Facial and Nasal Anatomy

Editor

SEBASTIAN COTOFANA

FACIAL PLASTIC SURGERY CLINICS OF NORTH AMERICA

www.facialplastic.theclinics.com

Consulting Editor
J. REGAN THOMAS

May 2022 • Volume 30 • Number 2

ELSEVIER

1600 John F. Kennedy Boulevard • Suite 1800 • Philadelphia, Pennsylvania, 19103-2899

http://www.theclinics.com

FACIAL PLASTIC SURGERY CLINICS OF NORTH AMERICA Volume 30, Number 2
May 2022 ISSN 1064-7406, ISBN-13: 978-0-323-84922-7

Editor: Stacy Eastman
Developmental Editor: Ann Gielou M. Posedio

Photocopying

Single photocopies of single articles may be made for personal use as allowed by national copyright laws. Permission of the Publisher and payment of a fee is required for all other photocopying, including multiple or systematic copying, copying for advertising or promotional purposes, resale, and all forms of document delivery. Special rates are available for educational institutions that wish to make photocopies for non-profit educational classroom use. For information on how to seek permission visit www.elsevier.com/permissions or call: (+44) 1865 843830 (UK)/ (+1) 215 239 3804 (USA).

Derivative Works

Subscribers may reproduce tables of contents or prepare lists of articles including abstracts for internal circulation within their institutions. Permission of the Publisher is required for resale or distribution outside the institution. Permission of the Publisher is required for all other derivative works, including compilations and translations (please consult www.elsevier.com/permissions).

Electronic Storage or Usage

Permission of the Publisher is required to store or use electronically any material contained in this periodical, including any article or part of an article (please consult www.elsevier.com/permissions). Except as outlined above, no part of this publication may be reproduced, stored in a retrieval system or transmitted in any form or by any means, electronic, mechanical, photocopying, recording or otherwise, without prior written permission of the Publisher.

Notice

No responsibility is assumed by the Publisher for any injury and/or damage to persons or property as a matter of products liability, negligence or otherwise, or from any use or operation of any methods, products, instructions or ideas contained in the material herein. Because of rapid advances in the medical sciences, in particular, independent verification of diagnoses and drug dosages should be made.

Although all advertising material is expected to conform to ethical (medical) standards, inclusion in this publication does not constitute a guarantee or endorsement of the quality or value of such product or of the claims made of it by its manufacturer.

Facial Plastic Surgery Clinics of North America (ISSN 1064-7406) is published quarterly by Elsevier Inc., 360 Park Avenue South, New York, NY 10010-1710. Months of issue are February, May, August, and November. Business and Editorial Offices: 1600 John F. Kennedy Blvd., Suite 1800, Philadelphia, PA 19103-2899. Periodicals postage paid at New York, NY, and additional mailing offices. Subscription prices are $420.00 per year (US individuals), $922.00 per year (US institutions), $468.00 per year (Canadian individuals), $950.00 per year (Canadian institutions), $557.00 per year (foreign individuals), $950.00 per year (foreign institutions), $100.00 per year (US students), $100.00 per year (Canadian students), and $255.00 per year (foreign students). Foreign air speed delivery is included in all *Clinics* subscription prices. All prices are subject to change without notice. POSTMASTER: Send address changes to *Facial Plastic Surgery Clinics*, Elsevier Health Sciences Division, Subscription Customer Service, 3251 Riverport Lane, Maryland Heights, MO 63043. **Customer service: 1-800-654-2452 (US and Canada); 1-314-447-8871 (outside US and Canada); Fax: 314-447-8029; E-mail: journalscustomerservice-usa@elsevier.com (for print support); journalsonlinesupport-usa@elsevier.com (for online support).**

Reprints. For copies of 100 or more of articles in this publication, please contact the Commercial Reprints Department, Elsevier Inc., 360 Park Avenue South, New York, NY 10010-1710. Tel.: 212-633-3874; Fax: 212-633-3820; E-mail: reprints@elsevier.com.

Facial Plastic Surgery Clinics of North America is covered in *MEDLINE/PubMed* (*Index Medicus*).

Contributors

CONSULTING EDITOR

J. REGAN THOMAS, MD
Professor, Facial Plastic and Reconstructive Surgery, Department of Otolaryngology–Head and Neck Surgery, Northwestern University Feinberg School of Medicine, Chicago, Illinois, USA

EDITOR

SEBASTIAN COTOFANA, MD, PhD
Anatomy Professor and Physician, Associate Professor of Anatomy, Department of Clinical Anatomy, Mayo Clinic College of Medicine and Science, Mayo Clinic, Rochester, Minnesota, USA

AUTHORS

MICHAEL G. ALFERTSHOFER
Medical Student, Department for Hand, Plastic and Aesthetic Surgery, University Hospital, Ludwig – Maximilian University Munich, Munich, Germany

HATEM AMER, MD
Division of Nephrology and Hypertension, Essam and Dalal Obaid Center for Reconstructive Transplant Surgery, William J. von Liebig Center for Transplantation and Clinical Regeneration, Mayo Clinic, Rochester, Minnesota, USA

SHIRIN ASSEMI-KABIR, DDS
Dentist, Department for Hand, Plastic and Aesthetic Surgery, Ludwig – Maximilian University Munich, Munich, Germany

KARIM BAKRI, MBBS
Division of Plastic Surgery, Department of Surgery, Mayo Clinic, Rochester, Minnesota, USA

FRANCESCO BERNARDINI, MD
Oculoplastica Bernardini, Genova, Italy

DAVID BRAIG, MD, PHD
Department for Hand, Plastic and Aesthetic Surgery, Ludwig – Maximilian University Munich, Munich, Germany

HALEY N. BRAY, MD
Fellow, Facial Plastic Surgery

NIKITA BREYER
Department of Hand, Plastic and Aesthetic Surgery, University Hospital, Ludwig – Maximilian University Munich, Munich, Germany

MIA CAJKOVSKY
Yuvell, Private Practice, Vienna, Austria

SEBASTIAN COTOFANA, MD, PhD
Anatomy Professor and Physician, Associate Professor of Anatomy, Department of Clinical Anatomy, Mayo Clinic College of Medicine and Science, Mayo Clinic, Rochester, Minnesota, USA

MIHAI DUMBRAVA, BS
Department of Clinical Anatomy, Mayo Clinic College of Medicine and Science, Rochester, Minnesota, USA

DENIS EHRL, MD, PhD
Physician, Department for Hand, Plastic and Aesthetic Surgery, Ludwig – Maximilian University Munich, Munich, Germany

KONSTANTIN FRANK, MD
Physician, Department for Hand, Plastic and Aesthetic Surgery, Ludwig – Maximilian University Munich, Munich, Germany

DAVID L. FREYTAG, MD
Department of Plastic Surgery, Community Hospital Havelhöhe, Berlin, Germany

LYSANDER FREYTAG, MD
Department of Plastic Surgery, Community Hospital Havelhöhe, Berlin, Germany

WALEED GIBREEL, MBBS
Division of Plastic Surgery, Department of Surgery, Mayo Clinic, Rochester, Minnesota, USA

RICCARDO E. GIUNTA, MD, PhD
Department for Hand, Plastic and Aesthetic Surgery, Ludwig – Maximilian University Munich, Munich, Germany

ROBERT H. GOTKIN, MD, FACS
Physician, Private Practice, New York, New York, USA

JEREMY B. GREEN, MD
Skin Associates of South Florida and Skin Research Institute, Coral Gables, Florida, USA

JOHN B. HARGISS, BS
Department of Clinical Anatomy, Mayo Clinic College of Medicine and Science, Rochester, Minnesota, USA

SABRINA HELM
Department for Hand, Plastic and Aesthetic Surgery, Ludwig – Maximilian University Munich, Munich, Germany

CLAUDIA A. HERNANDEZ, MD
Physician, CH Dermatologia, Medellin, Colombia

LUZI HOFMANN
Department of Hand, Plastic and Aesthetic Surgery, University Hospital, Ludwig – Maximilian University Munich, Munich, Germany

FABIO INGALLINA, MD
Private Practice, Catania, Italy

BENRITA JITAREE, PhD
Chakri Naruebodindra Medical Institute, Faculty of Medicine, Ramathibodi Hospital, Mahidol University, Samut Prakan, Thailand

RAMTIN KASSIR, MD
Park Avenue Plastic Surgery and Dermatology, Private Practice, New York, New York, USA

SHEILA KASSIR, MD
Park Avenue Plastic Surgery and Dermatology, Private Practice, New York, New York, USA

KONSTANTIN CHRISTOPH KOBAN, MD
Department of Hand, Plastic and Aesthetic Surgery, University Hospital, Ludwig – Maximilian University Munich, Munich, Germany

LUKAS H. KOHLER, MD
Department for Hand, Plastic and Aesthetic Surgery, Ludwig – Maximilian University Munich, Munich, Germany

ZHOUXIAO LI, MD
Department for Hand, Plastic and Aesthetic Surgery, Ludwig – Maximilian University Munich, Munich, Germany

PAUL Z. LORENC, MD
Physician, Private Practice, New York, New York, USA

FABIANO NADSON MAGACHO-VIEIRA, MD
Ceara State University, Department of Clinical, Aesthetic and Surgical Dermatology, Batista Memorial Hospital, Fortaleza, Ceará, Brazil

SAMIR MARDINI, MD
Professor and Chair, Division of Plastic and Reconstructive Surgery, Department of Surgery, Surgical Director, Essam and Dalal Obaid Center for Reconstructive Transplant Surgery, William J. von Liebig Center for Transplantation and Clinical Regeneration, Mayo Clinic, Rochester, Minnesota, USA

ARNALDO MERCADO-PEREZ, BS
Department of Clinical Anatomy, Mayo Clinic College of Medicine and Science, Rochester, Minnesota, USA

ELENA MILLESI
Division of Plastic and Reconstructive Surgery, Mayo Clinic, Rochester, Minnesota, USA

NICHOLAS MOELLHOFF, MD
Physician, Department for Hand, Plastic and Aesthetic Surgery, University Hospital, Ludwig

– Maximilian University Munich, Munich, Germany

AMANDA MOOREFIELD, BS
Medial Student, Kansas City University

TATJANA PAVICIC, MD
Physician, Private Practice, Munich, Germany

PHILIPP PERKO, MD
Department of Hand, Plastic and Aesthetic Surgery, University Hospital, Ludwig – Maximilian University Munich, Munich, Germany

THIRAWASS PHUMYOO, PhD
Department of Basic Medical Science, Faculty of Medicine Vajira Hospital, Navamindradhiraj University, Bangkok, Thailand

ALESSIO REDAELLI, MD
Private Practice, Milan, Italy

KENT REMINGTON, MD
Remington Laser Dermatology Centre, Calgary, Alberta, Canada

LEONIE SCHELKE, MD
Private Practice, Amsterdam, the Netherlands; Department of Dermatology, Erasmus MC, University Medical Centre, Rotterdam, the Netherlands

TIM STAIGER
Department for Hand, Plastic and Aesthetic Surgery, Ludwig – Maximilian University Munich, Munich, Germany

CHRISTOPHER C. SUREK, DO, FACS
Board Certified Plastic Surgeon, Surek Plastic Surgery, Assistant Professor of Anatomy, Kansas City University, Clinical Assistant Professor of Plastic Surgery, University of Kansas Medical Center

ARTHUR SWIFT, MD
Private Practice, Montreal, Quebec, Canada

JONATHAN M. SYKES, MD
Professor Emeritus, Facial Plastic Surgery, University of California, Davis Medical Center

PETER J. VELTHUIS, MD, PhD
Department of Dermatology, Erasmus MC, University Medical Centre, Rotterdam, the Netherlands

DARIA VOROPAI, MD
Private Practice, Amsterdam, the Netherlands

KRISHNA VYAS, MD, PhD, MHS
Division of Plastic Surgery, Department of Surgery, Mayo Clinic, Rochester, Minnesota, USA

JULIE WOODWARD, MD, PhD
Duke University Medical Center, Durham, North Carolina, USA

YA XU, MD
Department for Hand, Plastic and Aesthetic Surgery, Ludwig – Maximilian University Munich, Munich, Germany

Contents

> Understanding the relevance of anatomic and biomechanical principles is crucial when treating the face with soft tissue fillers to achieve a symmetric, soft, and natural-looking result while mitigating the risk of adverse events. The objective of this study is to summarize facial age-related effects, to relate them to facial biomechanics, and to establish guidelines for safe, effective, and esthetically pleasing full-face treatment following 3 basic principles while incorporating the latest scientific developments. This narrative review summarizes the current understanding of facial aging and its implications for facial biomechanics deduced from the authors' experience and research.

> Nonsurgical rhinoplasty procedures using soft tissue fillers have gained popularity. With the increasing frequency of such procedures, the incidence of intra-arterial injection of soft tissue filler material and subsequent ischemia has also risen. This article analyzes the topographic anatomy of the dorsal nasal artery in the nasal soft tissue to potentially enhance patient safety in nonsurgical rhinoplasty procedures. The dorsal nasal artery shows a variable topographic course, especially in relationship to the procerus muscle. By understanding the topographic courses of the dorsal nasal artery, aesthetic practitioners may be able to perform nonsurgical rhinoplasty procedures with increased safety and efficacy.

> The morphologic characteristics of Asian nose are a short or retracted columella, an acute nasolabial angle, and deficient tip projection. Both operative rhinoplasty and filler rhinoplasty have been used to improve the columellar angle and the tip of the nose in Asia. However, the possibility that complications may occur following aesthetic interventions from the vascular compromises at the columella, for example, skin necrosis, deformity, and blindness. Thus, it is crucial to operate the aesthetic approach by understanding the detailed configurations of the columellar artery that might help physicians minimize the chances of adverse events.

> Facial measurements serve as a valuable tool in the treatment planning of facial plastic surgery. The aim of this study was to evaluate the accuracy and reliability of standard 3D anthropometric measurements of the face made with one low-cost handheld 3D scanner and one industrial-type mobile 3D scanner. There are clear potential benefits of using 3D measurements by means of new handheld mobile scanners. However, the Sense scanner from the class of inexpensive scanners showed significant limitations in more complex areas such as the lip and nose, whereas proportions could be measured satisfactorily.

> Three-dimensional surface imaging (3DSI) has been shown to be a useful tool for plastic surgeons in the preoperative, intraoperative, and postoperative setting. The objective of this investigation was to compare the accuracy of facial surface distance measurements using both a handheld facial 3DSI device and a stationary whole-body 3DSI device. Users should be aware of deviations when obtaining 3DSI using the presented imaging devices but should not refrain from using them, as the absolute differences might be too small to play a role in both, clinical and research, settings.

> The demand for surgical and nonsurgical esthetic procedures in the nasal region has increased sharply in the past. Anatomic differences of the nose between different ethnicities need to be investigated thoroughly. The objective of this article is to analyze and compare morphometric features of the nose in a mixed Asian-Caucasian study population. The nasal length in Asians was statistically significantly greater than in Caucasians, also after having adjusted for facial height. The nasal dorsal bridge and the nasal base showed statistically significant differences. By keeping these anatomic differences in mind while treating patients, greater efficacy and safety can be achieved.

> Because of its central location in the face, the nose plays an important role in the aesthetic perception of the face. To improve the appearance of the nose, surgical and nonsurgical rhinoplasty techniques have been described, although it still

remains elusive if both options show comparable results in their aesthetic perception. This study assesses the fixation pattern and duration when looking at postinterventional images compared with baseline images for surgical and nonsurgical rhinoplasty procedures. According to this study, the nasal appearance, especially in a lateral view, is more fundamentally altered when surgical rhinoplasty is performed, compared with nonsurgical rhinoplasty.

> Facial transplantation is a vascularized composite allotransplantation, which may be considered in patients with extensive and challenging facial defects for which conventional reconstructive approaches fail to provide satisfactory functional and esthetic outcomes. Facial transplantation has the advantage of replacing defective or absent structures with anatomically identical tissues. Facial transplantation may provide functional, esthetic, and psychosocial benefits, but must be weighed against risks such as lifelong immunosuppression. Success is reliant on patient understanding, motivation, consent and compliance, and a multidisciplinary approach with careful team planning and organization. This review highlights the achievements, challenges, and future directions of this rapidly evolving field.

> This study investigated eye movement patterns using eye tracking technology when looking at preoperative and postoperative images of patients that underwent bilateral periorbital cosmetic surgery. The sequence of facial recognition before surgery was periorbital-nose-perioral, whereas following surgery it was nose-periorbital-perioral. This study revealed that the sequence of facial feature recognition is influenced by the aesthetic liking of the observer and that alteration to facial features influences the sequence of facial feature recognition. The eye movement pattern, however, seems to follow the internal representation of beauty where aesthetically pleasing facial features are observed later during first image exposure and are viewed shorter.

FACIAL PLASTIC SURGERY CLINICS OF NORTH AMERICA

SERIES OF RELATED INTEREST

Clinics in Plastic Surgery
https://www.plasticsurgery.theclinics.com
Otolaryngologic Clinics
https://www.oto.theclinics.com
Dermatologic Clinics
https://www.derm.theclinics.com

THE CLINICS ARE AVAILABLE ONLINE!
Access your subscription at:
www.theclinics.com

Foreword
Facial and Nasal Anatomy

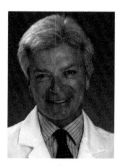

J. Regan Thomas, MD
Consulting Editor

A key area of expertise for those individuals whose medical and surgical practice is facial plastic and reconstructive surgery is an accurate knowledge of facial and nasal anatomy. Sebastian Cotofana, MD, PhD has been selected to be Guest Editor of this issue of *Facial Plastic Clinics of North America* due to his recognition as an excellent anatomist. Dr Cotofana has organized a unique and in-depth approach to discussing facial and nasal anatomy through a group of interesting and pertinent topics authored by outstanding experts in our field. Today's facial treatments entail an assortment of both surgical and nonsurgical treatments to provide superior results for the various patients' goals. Likewise, as this issue's contributing authors provide, there are multiple new methodologies to accurately investigate and demonstrate facial anatomy that can then be utilized in accurate treatment approaches.

In addition to relevant discussions of anatomic and facial appearance treatments, the authors also discuss appropriate and innovative anatomic evaluation modalities. The issue also discusses a variety of treatment techniques that benefit from these modern evaluation approaches. Useful modern methodologies that can be utilized are discussed, including ultrasound imaging, MRI, and computed tomographic scanning.

A wide spectrum of experienced and expert authors has been assembled to discuss and demonstrate the multiple components and insights to develop this issue. Key aspects of anatomy, facial function, and interesting aspects of clinical differences are discussed to create this interesting and unique issue, which will be of value to our readership.

J. Regan Thomas, MD
Facial Plastic and Reconstructive Surgery
Department of Otolaryngology–
Head and Neck Surgery
Northwestern University School of Medicine
60 East Delaware Place
Chicago, IL 60611, USA

E-mail address:
regan.thomas@nm.org

Facial Plast Surg Clin N Am 30 (2022) xiii
https://doi.org/10.1016/j.fsc.2022.03.016
1064-7406/22/© 2022 Published by Elsevier Inc.

Preface

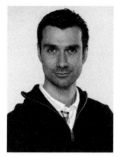

Sebastian Cotofana, MD, PhD
Editor

Dear colleagues,

It is my pleasure to serve as guest editor for this issue of *Facial Plastic Surgery Clinics of North America* dedicated to Facial and Nasal Anatomy. The demand for anatomic competence in facial anatomy has increased worldwide throughout the last few years. This is attributed not only to the emergence of various and novel surgical and nonsurgical facial procedures but also to the evolution of anatomy itself.

Despite that the word anatomy means literally "dissection" or "cutting apart," modern anatomy has little to do with such procedures. Of course, in medical school curricula and other allied health professions, learners still dissect by themselves or observe prosected human body donors to increase their anatomic competence. However, advancements in the medical field are obtained differently these days. Dissecting tissue is always associated with removing, detaching, opening, or changing the anatomic integrity of the area investigated. Once this happens, no original relationships can be appreciated anymore.

Therefore, new methodologies are utilized in anatomic research, like 3-dimensional surface scanning, ultrasound imaging, computed tomographic scanning, MRI, and ultrasound imaging. These methodologies are noninvasive visualization modalities that preserve the anatomic integrity for a better and functional understanding. This allowed for the introduction of a 3-dimensional understanding in today's facial procedures.

Anatomic research has also expanded from cadaveric research to clinical research, which was always a drawback when trying to extrapolate anatomic findings to daily clinical practice. With dedicated research, the field of facial biomechanics or injection biomechanics was established. These research domains are new and can be regarded as the fourth dimension of anatomic understanding. They add the factor time, that is, change over time or change during various facial movements, to the third dimension and allows for functional conclusions.

In this issue, friends and colleagues from all over the world have contributed with excellent articles to present facial and nasal anatomy utilizing up-to-date methodology presenting novel findings from the field of facial anatomy. I am sure you will this interesting and that this issue will increase your anatomic competence.

Best regards,
Sebastian Cotofana

Sebastian Cotofana, MD, PhD
Department of Clinical Anatomy
Mayo Clinic College of Medicine and Science
Rochester, MN 55905, USA

E-mail address:
Cotofana.Sebastian@mayo.edu

Facial Plast Surg Clin N Am 30 (2022) xv
https://doi.org/10.1016/j.fsc.2022.02.001
1064-7406/22/© 2022 Published by Elsevier Inc.

Understanding Facial Aging Through Facial Biomechanics

A Clinically Applicable Guide for Improved Outcomes

Lysander Freytag, MD[a,1], Michael G. Alfertshofer[b,1], Konstantin Frank, MD[b], Nicholas Moellhoff, MD[b], Sabrina Helm[b], Alessio Redaelli, MD[c], Daria Voropai, MD, DM[d], Claudia A. Hernandez, MD[e], Jeremy B. Green, MD[f], Sebastian Cotofana, MD, PhD[g,*]

KEYWORDS

- Facial aging • Facial biomechanics • Facial fat compartments • Fascial planes • Facial anatomy

INTRODUCTION

Facial aging is a multifactorial process that remains incompletely understood. Our current understanding summarizes the facial aging process as a series of continuous and intertwined events affecting all facial tissues, including bone, ligaments, muscles, fat, fasciae, and skin. These events begin at a variable age and progress at variable rates depending on the individual's gender, race, genetic footprint, and environmental exposure.[1–6] Although facial aging is an inevitable and irreversible process, its presentation on the skin surface can be influenced by a plethora of invasive and noninvasive procedures.[7–18] Of the variety of facial procedures available, minimally invasive soft tissue fillers have increased in popularity and acceptance when compared with other options like surgical interventions.[19]

Injectable soft tissue fillers are traditionally classified as volumizers and were introduced to the market to treat age-related volume loss. Recent research, however, has indicated that soft tissue fillers can be used to lift facial soft tissues (in addition to volumize them) when injected into dedicated facial regions and layers.[12,20] This development is novel and allows for the implementation of a variety of new treatment algorithms that increase effectiveness, safety, and patient satisfaction. Increased efficacy can be measured by the amount of product needed to achieve a desired esthetic outcome and/or by the longevity of the esthetic effect following the treatment. These effects have been demonstrated in clinical and cadaveric studies, and many of those principles have been widely adopted into daily practice.

However, to date, no comprehensive summary of those facial esthetic principles has been provided in the literature. By summarizing age-related events affecting various facial structures and relating them to the underlying biomechanics of the face, the authors hope to help injectors

Funding: This study received no funding.
[a] Department of Plastic Surgery, Community Hospital Havelhöhe, Berlin, Germany; [b] Department for Hand, Plastic and Aesthetic Surgery, Ludwig – Maximilian University Munich, Munich, Germany; [c] Private Practice, Milan, Italy; [d] Private Practice, Amsterdam, the Netherlands; [e] CH Dermatologia, Medellin, DC, USA; [f] Skin Associates of South Florida and Skin Research Institute, Coral Gables, FL, USA; [g] Department of Clinical Anatomy, Mayo Clinic College of Medicine and Science, Mayo Clinic, Stabile Building 9-38, 200 First Street, Rochester, MN 55905, USA
[1] Both authors contributed equally to this work.
* Corresponding author.
E-mail address: cotofana.sebastian@mayo.edu

Facial Plast Surg Clin N Am 30 (2022) 125–133
https://doi.org/10.1016/j.fsc.2022.01.001

better understand the rationale behind their treatments and to improve their techniques. The understanding of facial aging and facial biomechanics can enable injectors to see behind the curtain and to adjust their treatments to the individual needs of each patient rather than to follow rigid schemes and predefined injection algorithms. Personalizing treatments may increase procedural effectiveness and reduce treatment-related adverse events and therefore increase patient satisfaction.

Therefore, the objective of this anatomic narrative review is to summarize facial aging effects, relate them to facial biomechanics, and deduce guiding esthetic principles to enhance clinical practice.

METHODS

This narrative review summarizes the current understanding of facial aging and its implications for facial biomechanics. The views, conclusions, and treatment suggestions presented herein are the opinion of the authors and should be regarded as such.

FACIAL AGING
Facial Bones

Despite the general assumption that bones are static components of the skull, recent research has indicated that even the bones of the skull undergo age-related changes, which is termed bone remodeling.[6,21–23] Bone remodeling is the sum of multiple continuously ongoing changes in bone structure that influence bone shape. In the neurocranium, the calvaria is decreasing in its volume in both males and females, which results in the reduction in overall cranial volume.[4] This bone-related volume reduction influences the support for all overlying soft tissues resulting in less soft tissue support and stability. With bone-related volume reduction, facial soft tissues can follow the effects of gravity toward a more caudal position; this presents clinically as soft tissue descent.

In the midface, the viscerocranium likewise undergoes bone remodeling and primarily presents through the loss of the midfacial height.[6] The midfacial height was determined as the distance between the nasion and the nasal spine and was shown to decrease in height both in males and in females. This loss in midfacial height influences the overall bony support for the midfacial soft tissues, which contributes to the soft tissue descent observed during facial aging. In addition, the maxilla changes its anterior projection, which is reflected by the decrease in maxillary angle[24] again resulting in the loss of bony support for the overlying midfacial soft tissues.

In the lower face, the loss of alveolar height and dentition contributes to the loss of support for lower facial soft tissues including the lips and jowls, which is observed clinically as soft tissue descent.

Facial Ligaments

Facial ligaments are poorly understood, but the general concept is that they resemble true osteocutaneous connections that connect certain areas of the skin to the underlying bone. To date, there is no robust scientific evidence that with increasing age, facial ligaments increase in laxity and contribute therefore to the clinically observed facial soft tissue descent. It could be speculated that with bone remodeling and bone surface changes, the bony attachment of facial ligaments is concomitantly changing resulting in soft tissue effects that are (incorrectly) attributed to facial ligaments. Future studies will need to be designed to identify whether facial ligaments truly increase in laxity or if the observed facial soft tissue changes should be related to bone changes because ligaments are stable and unaffected by the influences of facial aging.

Facial Muscles

The muscles of facial expression are a specific type of musculature that allow for expression of emotions by moving the overlying skin. Almost all facial muscles have a direct connection to the bone and connect either with each other to form muscle complexes or attach to the skin to enable facial expressions. In certain facial areas the muscle fibers are directly connected to the dermal undersurface, and this tight interaction allows for minute movements of the overlying skin surface; this is needed especially in facial areas where precise movement is mandatory like the periorbital or perioral region. In other areas, facial muscles form complexes like the orbicularis oculi muscle complex, which has great relevance to neuromodulator injections, or like the orbicularis oris muscle complex, which is an important consideration during lip-volumizing procedures. The understanding of the anatomy of muscle complexes is crucial to guide and direct facial treatments because of the potential risk to affect other muscles in their close proximity: eyebrow elevators versus eyebrow depressors. Similar to the eyebrow, the (oral) modiolus is likewise at a balance between depressors (depressor anguli oris muscle, platysma, depressor labii inferioris) and elevators (levator anguli oris, zygomaticus major and minor, levator labii superioris) and their balance influences the position of the oral commissure and therefore lip position.

Recent research has indicated that age does not statistically significantly influence the signal-to-noise ratio (an adjusted electromyographic parameter) when comparing young versus old individuals in a large sampled study.[25] However, subanalyses have indicated that the signal increases in the corrugator supercilii and procerus muscles potentially explaining why glabellar rhytides are more prominent with increasing age. In addition, the same study revealed that the zygomaticus major muscle decreases in its signal in older patients potentially indicating a reduced motor unit action potential of this muscle. This age-related effect of the zygomaticus major was similarly observed in a previous independent ultrasound-based investigation in which researchers found that the ability to compress the angular vein against the underlying maxilla is reduced in individuals of older age when compared with a younger cohort of their sample.[26]

Facial Fat

Facial fat is arranged in 2 parallel layers of fat, which is separated by the superficial fascia of the face and is termed superficial musculoaponeurotic system (SMAS) in the middle face. Although both fatty layers have been shown to be compartmentalized,[27–33] a previous study has revealed that the superficial fat compartments can descend during the process of facial aging,[3] whereas the deep fat compartments do not change in their position relative to the underlying bone.[2] This increased mobility of the superficial fat compartments explains why with increasing age the nasolabial sulcus becomes more prominent, as do the jowls and the labiomandibular sulcus.

With increasing age, the overall facial fat mass reduces independent of the body mass index of the investigated person resulting in decreased facial soft tissue thickness.[7–9] If facial fat is understood as the material located inside facial compartments, its age-related reduction can cause the walls of the respective compartments to have reduced structural stability. A reduced structural stability can favor facial soft tissue descent following the effects of gravity.

Facial Fascias

The fascias of the face are separating and dividing structures that either connect structures to the underlying bone (= facial vein canal) or that separate facial layers from each other (= SMAS). In the face, a superficial fascia (separation between superficial

and deep fat compartments) and a deep fascia can be identified, the latter being variable in presence and extent. In the tear trough, for instance, no deep fascia can be identified. The facial SMAS is not a single, flat layer of connective tissue but a 3-dimensional composite of fat and fibrous collagenous tissue. The SMAS serves to transmit the movement of the underlying facial muscles to the overlying skin by incorporating some facial muscles like the zygomaticus major. Recent research has also indicated that the SMAS itself contains muscle fibers,[34] providing an explanatory model for the effectiveness of microtoxin treatments.

Facial fascias connect various facial tissues, and the superficial fascia in particular has been shown to be a continuous layer enveloping the entire cranium. In the scalp it is termed galea aponeurotica, in the temple superficial temporal fascia, in the forehead it is represented by the frontalis muscle, in the periorbital region by the orbicularis oculi muscle, in the midface it is termed SMAS, and in the lateral lower face it is termed platysma. Age-related effects of facial fascias have to date not been investigated in detail.

FACIAL BIOMECHANICS
General Descriptions

The classic understanding of biomechanical concepts, that is, the movement of living tissue is also applicable to the human face despite the fact that it is poorly investigated and understood. The observed facial movements are primarily effected by the muscles of facial expression and by the muscles of mastication (eye and tongue movements excluded), both of which are classified as striated muscles.[35,36] The muscles of mastication are exclusively located in the lateral face, whereas the muscles of facial expression are predominately located in the medial face, that is, the central facial oval. Movements of the face are not classified according to the standard descriptions of flexion/extension or abductions/adduction but in relation to the respective facial expression: smiling, frowning, and so forth.

Line of Ligaments

Facial movements are different in the medial versus the lateral face due to the presence of the line of ligaments.[37] The line of ligaments is a linear surface landmark that extends from the temple to the mandible and is the surface projection of 4 of the most relevant facial ligaments: temporal ligamentous adhesion, lateral orbital thickening, zygomatic ligament, and mandibular ligament. A recent study has revealed that the movement in the medial face is directed laterally, whereas the movement of the lateral face is directed medially converging at the line of ligaments, indicating that the line of ligaments is not only a surface landmark but also a functional boundary between the medial and the lateral face. The difference in movement between the medial and the lateral face, and the incorporation of these line-related differences into treatment algorithms, has been revealed to result in superior outcomes.[38,39]

Fascial Arrangement

In the medial midface, the fascial arrangement of facial soft tissues Is oblique due to the presence of facial muscles. Almost all facial muscles originate from the bone and insert into the overlying skin or other superficially located muscle complexes indicating an oblique course, that is, from deep to superficial. This oblique fascial arrangement includes the presence of encapsulated superficial and deep fat compartments, which fill the spaces between the oblique fascial layers. As a consequence soft tissue filler injections in the medial result predominately in surface projection, that is, volumization. In the lateral face, the fascial layers are arranged in parallel layers without the presence of muscles of facial expression and without the presence of deep facial fat compartments. Owing to the absence of major facial ligaments in the lateral face, no strong connection to the underlying bone or deep fascia is possible, allowing the lateral facial soft tissue to be majorly affected by gravity and age-related facial soft tissue descent. The latter is additionally influenced by the fact that all layers are connected with each other as they extend from the scalp to the neck enabling lower facial components to pull upper facial components inferiorly.

Facial Mobility: Medial versus Lateral Face

Owing to the presence of facial muscles in the medial face (and not in the lateral face), the medial face is also termed the mobile face. However, this term needs to be interpreted with caution because the mobility observed in the medial face is *active* mobility, which is aff"ected by the muscles of facial expression. In the lateral face, however, no facial muscles can be found, which explains why active mobility (apart from movements of the temporomandibular joint) is absent here. However, unpublished data (Freytag, 2021) have indicated that *passive* mobility, which is predominantly affected by gravity and age-related changes, is increased in the lateral face when compared with the medial face. Experiments with healthy volunteers have indicated that during postural changes (from standing upright to lying down) the lateral face

displays greater mobility than the medial face. This greater mobility is plausible because in the lateral face there is no major direct connection to the underlying deep fascia or bone and there is an absence of facial muscles and major facial ligaments.

Facial Mobility: Superficial versus Deep

During facial movements the underlying soft tissues glide over deeper structures. Cadaveric studies have provided evidence that the deep fat compartments do not glide in relation to the underlying bone but have a stable location during facial expressions like smiling or during the process of facial aging[2,40]; this is plausible because the boundaries of those compartments are formed by muscular, ligamentous, or fascial bony connections, which are stable, and their bony connections are not affected by the process of facial aging. In contrast, the superficial fat compartments have been revealed to display greater mobility than the deep compartments during facial expressions (like smiling) or during a simulated aging process[40]; this is likewise feasible when accepting that the muscles of facial expression travel from deep to superficial and while being incorporated and connected to the SMAS they can move the superficial fat compartments substantially. The SMAS is a 3-dimensional compound consisting of connective tissue and the superficial fat compartments, and its movement will influence the position of the superficial fat compartments in relation to the underlying bone. Additional evidence for the increased mobility of the superficial fat compartments has been provided by the first description of the transverse facial septum and the overfilled syndrome.[41] Here, researchers have demonstrated that during smiling the medial midfacial volume increases (clinically termed: apple cheeks formation), which is affected by the contraction of the transverse facial septum due to its conformational change and the resulting cranial displacement of the compartments residing in this fascial hammock.

Resulting Principles for Soft Tissue Filler Injections

Based on the effects of facial aging in interplay with the biomechanical concepts of facial movements, several principles for soft tissue filler treatments can be elucidated. These principles could guide injectors of all skill levels in designing and implementing treatment algorithms. These algorithms would respect the effects of the aging process and include the biomechanical soft tissue movements.

First Principle: Upper Face First

During the process of facial aging, myriad changes occur in all facial tissues and layers. However, the end result of these processes is soft tissue descent following the effects of gravity. Bone remodeling results in loss of support for overlying soft tissues; facial fat decreases in volume, which results in reduced content of superficial and deep fat compartments; some muscles of facial expression display less motor unit action potential resulting in less muscular support against the effects of gravity; and facial ligaments and fascias do not limit the gliding of the overlying soft tissues especially in the lateral face, thus permitting soft tissue descent from the upper face to the lower face.

Starting full face treatments in the upper face or in the region above the facial region of esthetic interest would allow one to reposition the facial soft tissues approximating their original location and to prevent further soft tissue descent. Recent research has revealed that injecting soft tissue fillers of high viscoelastic properties into the subdermal plane of the superior temple can reduce midfacial volume and accentuate the contour of the jawline by repositioning the lateral facial soft tissues[42]; this has subsequently been confirmed in several independent clinical and cadaveric investigations, which have resulted in the development of the temporal lifting technique.

The *upper face first* principle can be also applied to the medial midface, which is the current standard clinical practice (**Fig. 1**). The need for filler

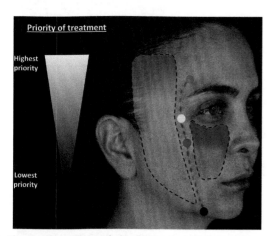

Fig. 1. Illustration of the first principle "upper face first" in a female patient. The color gradients indicate the chronology of injections in the respective area. According to this principle, the first injection in the lateral face (blue area) should be placed cranially in the temple region, followed by subsequent injections more caudally. This injection sequence (from cranial to caudal) also applies to the medial midface (*red area*) where cranial aspects should be injected first.

injections directly into the nasolabial fold is often obviated by first volumizing the upper midface, that is, the prezygomatic space of the suborbicularis oculi fat.

Starting a full face treatment in the lower face would increase the absolute weight of the lower facial soft tissues due to the filler application and would result in unnatural outcomes if the tissues are volumized a priori without repositioning. It should be noted that the loss in volume originates from the inferior repositioning (descent) of the soft tissues and subsequent unmasking of the remainder of the soft tissue volume deficit in the upper and/or middle face. A clinical example is the palpebromalar groove in the lateral infraorbital area. The groove is visible due to the descent of the midfacial soft tissues that unmask the inferior orbital rim. Current treatment strategies volumize the midface inferior to the groove and therefore reposition the midfacial soft tissues to cover (again) the exposed inferior orbital rim.

Second Principle: Lateral Face First

The lateral face is separated from the medial face by a functional boundary formed by the line of ligaments.[43] This functional boundary also corresponds to the change in layered arrangement of the fascial layers with a parallel arrangement laterally and an oblique arrangement medially. The oblique arrangement medially has no effect in the adjacent facial regions: treatments of the forehead cannot influence the medial midface due to the presence of the eyes and the medial midface cannot influence the perioral region due to the presence to the mouth. However, the lateral facial layers extend into the medial face with the SMAS being connected to the superficial temporal fascia, to the orbicularis oculi, and to the platysma.

Injections of soft tissue fillers following the *lateral face first* principle have been clinically shown to precondition the medial midface and to result in less product volume usage to achieve a symmetric outcome in a split-face study.[39] Product administration in the lateral face first, that is, targeting areas lateral to the line of ligaments first, can reposition the medial facial soft tissues due to the fascial connection from lateral to medial (**Fig. 2**). Targeting the medial facial regions first would influence the lateral facial regions only to a limited extent due to the characteristics of medial midfacial treatments, which result predominantly in volumizing and not in soft tissue repositioning.

Treating midfacial volume loss is currently the standard clinical practice to address by injecting the medial zygomatic and lateral infraorbital regions first and then to volumize the midface if

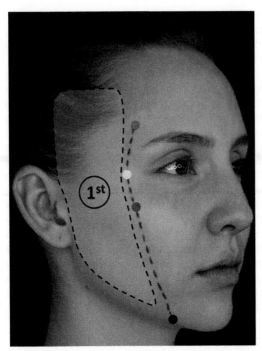

Fig. 2. Illustration of the second principle "lateral face first" in a female patient. The medial border of the lateral face is the "line of ligaments," an imaginary line connecting relevant ligamentous structures.[38]

needed. In addition, midfacial volume deficiency needs to be assessed and addressed with dynamic facial filling due to the presence of the transverse facial septum. Applying soft tissue fillers in the midface without controlling for the effect of upper midfacial volume increase during various facial expressions can result clinically in the facial over-filled syndrome.[13,41] Here a normal to high volume is observed at rest, but during smiling an exaggerated volume can be detected in the midface following the cranial displacement of the midfacial fat compartments.

Third Principle: Deep Injections First

The deep facial fat compartments have been shown to displace less during the process of facial aging and to move less during facial animation when controlled in vivo with ultrasound analyses[40]; this is plausible because their boundaries are connected to the underlying bone, and this connection is not affected by age or facial animation. The superficial fat compartments, however, have been shown to descend during facial aging and to display statistically significant greater movement when compared with the deep facial fat compartments.

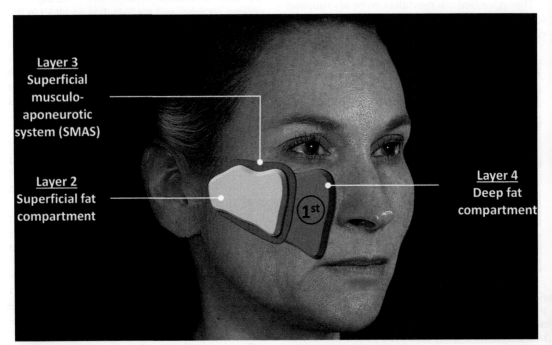

Fig. 3. Illustration of the third principle "deep injections first" in a female patient. According to this principle, injections into the deep fat compartments can help build a fundament for the overlying superficial soft tissues of the face. The deep fat compartment (layer 4) is separated by the superficial musculoaponeurotic system (SMAS, layer 3) from the superficial fat compartment.

Targeting the deep planes, that is, the supraperiosteal planes first following the principle *deep injection first* would allow the injector to re-create the bony fundament and to build support for the mobile overlying facial soft tissues (**Fig. 3**); this would potentially enable the more superficially located soft tissues to reposition and also to glide and move freely and naturally with facial expressions without interference of the soft tissue filler. Targeting the superficial fat compartments first can result in a less natural facial appearance with movement. The fat compartment cranially to the nasolabial sulcus is not targeted a priori because it is known to worsen the appearance of the fold; similarly the jowls fat compartment is not targeted with soft tissue fillers because it has been observed to worsen the appearance of the labiomandibular sulcus and the jowls deformity. An additional benefit to treating deep first is that in general fine-etched rhytides in the skin are present over areas of deeper volume deficit. In the authors' experience, volumizing these sites deeply (supraperiosteal and subcutaneous) results in improvement of fine lines, thus requiring less superficial (intradermal) injected volume and esthetically more pleasing outcomes.

This principle is also pertinent for soft tissue filler injection safety.[44] Recent investigations have revealed that the supraperiosteal plane of the face is in general a safer plane to administer soft tissue fillers because the facial arterial vasculature travels in more superficial planes (with regional exceptions).

SUMMARY

Understanding the individual changes of facial soft tissues that contribute to the overarching process termed facial aging is challenging. The resulting effect, however, facial soft tissue descent, is understandable in the context of facial biomechanics. To date no scientific report has summarized and combined both facial concepts (facial aging and facial biomechanics) to delineate principles for soft tissue filler injections. The 3 principles presented herein are not in and of themselves novel because they are performed on a relatively regular basis in clinical practice. The presented work, however, does distill the current available knowledge into 3 principles, which hopefully will guide practitioners toward increasing efficiency when ameliorating the signs of facial aging. Nevertheless, individualized treatments following patient assessment in combination with the esthetic desires of the patient will require adaptation and customization of the learnings presented herein.

CLINICS CARE POINTS

- First principle "Upper face first": With increasing age, the soft tissues descend. By starting minimally-invasive aesthetic full face treatments in the upper face/above the region of aesthetic interest, the soft tissues can be repositioned in their original location.
- Second principle "Lateral face first": Injecting soft tissue fillers into the lateral face (i.e. lateral to the "line of ligaments") first can precondition the medial face by repositioning its soft tissues ultimately leading to more effective treatments while simultaneously using less product.
- Third principle "Deep injections first": According to this principle, soft tissue filler material should ideally be placed in the deep plane (i.e. supraperiosteal) first. Due to the connections to the underlying bone, deep facial fat compartments have been shown to move less during facial animation compared to the superficial fat compartments. Injecting soft tissue filler material into the deep plane would allow for a strengthening of the bony fundament of the overlying facial soft tissues.

AUTHOR DISCLOSURE

None of the authors listed have any commercial associations or financial disclosures that might pose or create a conflict of interest with the methods applied or the results presented in this article.

REFERENCES

1. Fratila A, Schenck T, Redka-Swoboda W, et al. The anatomy of the aging face: a review. Facial Plast Surg 2016;32(03):253–60.
2. Cotofana S, Gotkin RH, Frank K, et al. The functional anatomy of the deep facial fat compartments: a detailed imaging-based investigation. Plast Reconstr Surg 2019;143:53–63.
3. Schenck TL, Koban KC, Schlattau A, et al. The functional anatomy of the superficial fat compartments of the face: a Detailed Imaging Study. Plast Reconstr Surg 2018;141:1351–9.
4. Cotofana S, Gotkin RH, Ascher B, et al. Calvarial volume loss and facial aging: a computed tomographic (CT)-Based Study. Aesthet Surg J 2018;38:1043–51.
5. Frank K, Gotkin RH, Pavicic T, et al. Age and gender differences of the frontal bone: a computed

tomographic (ct)-based Study. Aesthet Surg J 2018; 39(7):699–710.

6. Cotofana S, Gotkin RH, Morozov SP, et al. The relationship between bone remodeling and the clockwise rotation of the facial skeleton. Plast Reconstr Surg 2018;142(6):1447–54.

7. Sepe A, Tchkonia T, Thomou T, et al. Aging and regional differences in fat cell progenitors - A mini-review. Gerontology 2010;57:66–75.

8. Palmer AK, Kirkland JL. Aging and adipose tissue: potential interventions for diabetes and regenerative medicine. Exp Gerontol 2016;86:97–105.

9. Lakowa N, Trieu N, Flehmig G, et al. Telomere length differences between subcutaneous and visceral adipose tissue in humans. Biochem Biophys Res Commun 2015;457:426–32.

10. Lefebvre-Vilardebo M, Trevidic P, Moradi A, et al. Hand: Clinical anatomy and regional approaches with injectable fillers. Plast Reconstr Surg 2015; 136(5 Suppl):258S–75S.

11. Braz A, Humphrey S, Weinkle S, et al. Lower face: clinical anatomy and regional approaches with injectable fillers. Plast Reconstr Surg 2015;136: 235S–57S.

12. Haidar R, Freytag DL, Frank K. Quantitative analysis of the lifting effect of facial soft-tissue filler injections. Plast Reconstr Surg 2021;147(5):765e–76e.

13. Cotofana S, Schenck TL, Trevidic P, et al. Midface: clinical anatomy and regional approaches with injectable fillers. Plast Reconstr Surg 2015;136:219S–34S.

14. Sykes JM, Cotofana S, Trevidic P, et al. Upper face: clinical anatomy and regional approaches. Plast Reconstr Surg 2015;136:204S–18S.

15. Song A, Askari M, Azemi E, et al. Biomechanical properties of the superficial fascial system. Aesthet Surg J 2006;26(4):395–403.

16. MacGregor JL, Tanzi EL. Microfocused ultrasound for skin tightening. Semin Cutan Med Surg 2013; 32:18–25.

17. Dayan SH, Arkins JP, Chaudhry R. Minimally invasive neck lifts: have they replaced neck lift surgery? Facial Plast Surg Clin North Am 2013;21:265–70.

18. Gold MH, Biesman BS, Taylor M. Enhanced high-energy protocol using a fractional bipolar radiofrequency device combined with bipolar radiofrequency and infrared light for improving facial skin appearance and wrinkles. J Cosmet Dermatol 2017;16:205–9.

19. Global Statistics Report 2019 - Internation Society of Aesthetic Plastic Surgery (Accessed 02 February 2022), 2019.

20. Suwanchinda A, Webb KL, Rudolph C, et al. The posterior temporal supraSMAS minimally invasive lifting technique using soft-tissue fillers. J Cosmet Dermatol 2018;17:617–24.

21. Karunanayake M, To F, Efanov JI, et al. Analysis of craniofacial remodeling in the aging midface using

reconstructed three-dimensional models in paired individuals. Plast Reconstr Surg 2017;140:448e–54e.

22. Pessa JE, Desvigne LD, Lambros VS, et al. Changes in ocular globe-to-orbital rim position with age: implications for aesthetic blepharoplasty of the lower eyelids. Aesthetic Plast Surg 1999;23(5):337–42.

23. Kim SJ, Kim SJ, Park JS, et al. Analysis of age-related changes in asian facial skeletons using 3D vector mathematics on picture archiving and communication system computed tomography. Yonsei Med J 2015;56(5):1395.

24. Pessa JE. An algorithm of facial aging: Verification of Lambros's theory by three-dimensional stereolithography, with reference to the pathogenesis of midfacial aging, scleral show, and the lateral suborbital trough deformity. Plast Reconstr Surg 2000;106(2):479–88.

25. Cotofana S, Assemi-Kabir S, Mardini S, et al. Understanding Facial Muscle Aging: A Surface Electromyography Study. Aesthet Surg J 2021;41(9):NP1208–17.

26. Cotofana S, Lowry N, Devineni A, et al. Can smiling influence the blood flow in the facial vein?—An experimental study. J Cosmet Dermatol 2020;19: 321–7.

27. Gierloff M, Stöhring C, Buder T, et al. The subcutaneous fat compartments in relation to aesthetically important facial folds and rhytides. J Plast Reconstr Aesthet Surg 2012;65:1292–7.

28. Cotofana S, Schenck TL, Trevidic P, et al. Midface: clinical anatomy and regional approaches. Plast Reconstr Surg 2015;136:219S–34S.

29. Pilsl U, Anderhuber F. The chin and adjacent fat compartments. Dermatol Surg 2010;36(2):214–8.

30. Pilsl U, Anderhuber F. The septum subcutaneum parotideomassetericum. Dermatol Surg 2010;36(12): 2005–8.

31. Rohrich RJ, Pessa JE. The fat compartments of the face: anatomy and clinical implications for cosmetic surgery. Plast Reconstr Surg 2007;119(7):2219–27.

32. Reece EM, Pessa JE, Rohrich RJ. The mandibular septum: anatomical observations of the jowls in aging-implications for facial rejuvenation. Plast Reconstr Surg 2008;121(4):1414–20.

33. Garcia De Mitchell CA, Pessa JE, Schaverien MV, et al. The philtrum: anatomical observations from a new perspective. Plast Reconstr Surg 2008;122(6): 1756–60.

34. Sandulescu T, Weniger J, Philippou S, et al. Immunohistochemical evidence of striated muscle cells within midfacial superficial musculoaponeurotic system. Ann Anat 2021;234:151647.

35. Marur T, Tuna Y, Demirci S. Facial anatomy. Clin Dermatol 2014;32(1):14–23.

36. Ito J, Moriyama H, Shimada K. Morphological evaluation of the human facial muscles. Okajimas Folia Anat Jpn 2006;83(1):7–14.

37. Freytag DL, Alfertshofer MG, Frank K, et al. The difference in facial movement between the medial and

the lateral midface: a 3-dimensional skin surface vector analysis. Aesthet Surg J 2021;42(1):1–9.

38. Casabona G, Bernardini FP, Skippen B, et al. How to best utilize the line of ligaments and the surface volume coefficient in facial soft tissue filler injections. J Cosmet Dermatol 2020;19:303–11.

39. Casabona G, Frank K, Koban KC, et al. Lifting vs volumizing-The difference in facial minimally invasive procedures when respecting the line of ligaments. J Cosmet Dermatol 2019;18(5):1237–43.

40. Schelke L, Velthuis PJ, Lowry N, et al. The Mobility of the superficial and deep midfacial fat compartments – an ultrasound – based investigation. J Cosmet Dermatol 2021;20(12):3849–56.

41. Cotofana S, Gotkin RH, Frank K, et al. Anatomy behind the facial overfilled syndrome: The transverse facial septum. Dermatol Surg 2020;46(8): e16–22.

42. Hernandez CA, Freytag DL, Gold MH, et al. Clinical validation of the temporal lifting technique using soft tissue fillers. J Cosmet Dermatol 2020;19(10):2529–35.

43. Cotofana S, Lachman N. Anatomy of the Facial Fat Compartments and their Relevance in Aesthetic Surgery. J Dtsch Dermatol Ges 2019;17:399–413.

44. Freytag DL, Frank K, Haidar R, et al. Facial safe zones for soft tissue filler injections: a practical guide. J Drugs Dermatol 2019;18:896–902.

Ultrasound Anatomy of the Dorsal Nasal Artery as it Relates to Liquid Rhinoplasty Procedures

Michael G. Alfertshofer[a], Konstantin Frank, MD[a], Nicholas Moellhoff, MD[a], Sabrina Helm[a], Lysander Freytag, MD[b], Arnaldo Mercado-Perez, BS[c], John B. Hargiss, BS[c], Mihai Dumbrava, BS[c], Jeremy B. Green, MD[d], Sebastian Cotofana, MD, PhD[c],*

KEYWORDS

- Nasal anatomy • Dorsal nasal artery • Fascial layers • Soft tissue filler injections • Adverse events

INTRODUCTION

In 2020 according to statistics released by the Aesthetic Society a total of 55,436 surgical rhinoplasty procedures were performed in the United States generating revenue of more than $250 million.[1] Whereas severe and reconstructive cases require surgical intervention, small nasal profile changes have been shown to be amenable to minimally invasive soft tissue filler injections resulting in high patient satisfaction.[2–5] Although various injection techniques are available using either needles or cannulas, the safety of such procedures has been questioned based on recent reports of severe arterial vascular events including vision loss.[6]

The currently accepted pathomechanism behind such catastrophic sequelae is the injection of soft tissue filler material into the arterial blood, which is then transported to the ophthalmic artery circulation.[7] The latter provides the major blood supply to the retinal layers via the short, long, and posterior ciliary and central retinal arteries.[8] Obstruction caused by the filler material itself or

by the induced thrombus can cause irreversible damage to the supplied tissue resulting in vision loss.[9] Injecting the nasal soft tissues with volumizing soft tissue filler material carries such risk for several reasons: there is minimal soft tissue thickness of the nasal dorsum, which allows little space for the needle/cannula to glide around the artery; the nasal soft tissues have limited flexibility, which restricts the in situ mobility of the arteries if a needle/cannula is advanced against the arterial wall; and the arteries are directly connected to the ophthalmic artery circulation via the dorsal nasal artery (DNA), the lateral nasal artery, and the terminal branches of the anterior ethmoidal artery.[8,10–12]

To mitigate the risk of adverse events, the authors recommend that injectors familiarize themselves with the anatomy of the nasal layers and arterial vasculature.[13] Most of the literature addressing nasal soft tissue anatomy and its respective arterial vasculature involves investigations conducted in Asian populations or Asian body donors.[14–18] It is unclear whether these results can be extrapolated to Whites, including

Funding: This study received no funding.
[a] Department for Hand, Plastic and Aesthetic Surgery, Ludwig-Maximilian University Munich, Germany; [b] Department of Plastic Surgery, Community Hospital Havelhöhe, Berlin, Germany; [c] Department of Clinical Anatomy, Mayo Clinic College of Medicine and Science, Rochester, MN, USA; [d] Skin Associates of South Florida and Skin Research Institute, Coral Gables, FL, USA
* Corresponding author. Department of Clinical Anatomy, Mayo Clinic College of Medicine and Science, Mayo Clinic, Stabile Building 9-38, 200 First Street, Rochester, MN, 55905.
E-mail address: cotofana.sebastian@mayo.edu

arterial vascular variations and nasal soft tissue anatomy. In addition, most studies to ascertain tissue relationships/measurements were conducted on body donors, which may be considered a limitation.

The objective of this study is to investigate in a large White cohort the soft tissue relationship, the location, and the variation of the DNA by noninvasive ultrasound imaging as it relates to liquid rhinoplasty procedures. Using ultrasound imaging as the methodology of choice allows for measurements conducted in living subjects and without tissue disruption inherent in anatomic dissections. The underlying layered anatomy is visualized, and the arterial vasculature is measured and classified transcutaneously. It is hoped that the results of this study expand on and confirm previous studies conducted in Asian ethnicities and allow them to be generalizable to the White community without the use of a cadaveric model.

MATERIALS AND METHODS
Study Sample

Fifty-one healthy White volunteers (27 men, 24 women) were included in this investigation. The mean age was 29.31 (12.1) years (range, 19–63) and mean body mass index (BMI) was 23.42 (3.4) kg/m^2 (range, 17.6–34.3). Volunteers were recruited by the Department for Hand, Plastic and Aesthetic Surgery, Ludwig-Maximilian University Munich (Munich, Germany). Each volunteer provided written informed consent for the use of their data and associated images before their initiation into the study. The study was approved by the Institutional Review Board of Ludwig-Maximilian University Munich (protocol number: 19–999). This study was conducted in accordance with regional laws in Germany and good clinical practice.

Volunteers were not included in this analysis if they previously had undergone any type of corrective or reconstructive surgery or if they had any type of soft tissue filler injection performed on their nose.

Ultrasound Imaging

Volunteers were seated in an upright (45°) position during the ultrasound imaging of their nose. An 18-MHz linear transducer (LOGIQ S7 Expert, GE Healthcare GmbH, Solingen, Germany) was used for all imaging procedures that were performed by the same investigator (MA) to ensure consistency throughout measurements. The use of ultrasound contact gel (Aquasonic® Clear Ultrasound Gel, Parker Laboratories Inc, Fairfield, NJ) enabled the visualization of nasal layers and of the DNA

without direct skin contact; this allowed for accurate soft tissue measurements without compression.

The following parameters were evaluated:

- Total soft tissue thickness at the location of the DNA (absolute and percent) (**Fig. 1**)
- Distance between the DNA and the skin surface (see **Fig. 1**)
- Distance between the DNA and the nasal periosteum (see **Fig. 1**)
- Distance between the dorsal nasal anastomosis and the nasal radix (**Figs. 2 and 3**)
- Diameter of the DNA measured in the nasal midline
- Relationship between DNA and procerus muscle (**Figs. 4 and 5**)

Statistical Analysis

Descriptive analyses, bivariate correlations, and gender differences using independent Student t test were calculated using SPSS Statistics version 23 (IBM, Armonk, NY) and differences were considered statistically significant at a probability level of less than or equal to 0.05 to guide conclusions.

RESULTS
General Observations

The women in this study had a statistically significantly lower BMI compared with men (21.54 [2.7] kg/m^2 vs 25.10 [3.1] kg/m^2) with P less than 0.001 indicating an overall thinner soft tissue thickness; no such differences were detected when comparing gender-related differences for age ($P = .486$).

Depth and Diameter of Dorsal Nasal Artery

The total soft tissue thickness at the location of the DNA was 4.06 ± 0.5 mm in women and 4.81 ± 0.7 mm in men ($P < .001$). A statistically significant positive correlation was detected between the total soft tissue thickness and the BMI of study volunteers ($r_p = .535$; $P < .001$), indicating that a higher BMI increases the overall nasal soft tissue thickness.

The distance between skin surface and the DNA was in women 2.43 ± 0.4 mm and in men 2.75 ± 0.5 mm ($P < .018$; overall range of 1.70–3.80 mm independent of gender). The distance between the DNA and the nasal periosteum was 1.63 ± 0.6 mm in women and 2.07 ± 0.6 in men ($P = .014$ with an overall range of 0.90–3.30 mm independent of gender). This results in a relative depth (percentage, in relation to the total soft tissue thickness) of 60.5 ± 11.0% in females and of

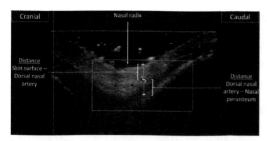

Fig. 1. Doppler-supported ultrasound image showing the distance measurements related to the DNA. The upper measurement shows the distance between skin surface and the artery. The lower measurement shows the distance between the artery and the nasal periosteum. The total nasal soft tissue thickness in the location of the DNA is the sum of both values.

57.6 ± 8.8% in males (*P* = .381) without statistically significant relationship to the BMI of the study volunteers (*P* = .072).

The diameter of the DNA was 0.6 ± 0.2 mm without statistically significant difference between genders (*P* = 1.00).

Location of Dorsal Nasal Artery

The anastomosis of the DNA with the contralateral side in the midline was located at an average distance of 5.61 ± 1.7 mm in women and 7.95 ± 3.5 mm in men inferior to the nasal radix (*P* = .009). The distance between radix and the DNA was not statistically correlated to the total length of the nose (r_p = .058; *P* = .711), indicating that the location of the DNA is influenced by other factors than the nasal length.

The DNA was identified to have a variable location in relationship to the procerus muscle, which originates from the nasal bone in close proximity to the osteochondral fusion (= rhinion). In women, the DNA was mainly (62.5%; n = 15) located deep to the procerus muscle, whereas in men it was predominantly (77.7%; n = 21) located superficial

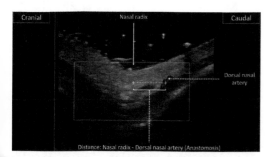

Fig. 2. Doppler-supported ultrasound image showing the distance measurement between the nasal radix and the anastomosis of the DNAs of both sides in the midline.

to the procerus muscle, a statistically significant difference between genders (*P* = .005). Overall, the DNA was more frequently identified superficial to the procerus muscle (58.8%; n = 30) than deep to the muscle (41.2%; n = 21).

DISCUSSION

This study was designed to evaluate whether previous studies conducted in Asian populations were applicable to the White community by using noninvasive ultrasound imaging in a large cohort (n = 51). The results revealed that the thickness of nasal soft tissues when measured in the location of the DNA statistically significantly correlated with the BMI of the study participants with higher BMI values being related to greater soft tissue thickness (r_p = .535; *P* < .001). This is plausible because the increase in BMI concomitantly increases the thickness of the subcutaneous fatty layer, which is also present at the dorsum of the nose and can therefore increase the local thickness. This in turn indicates that absolute values presented for nasal soft tissue thickness needs to be adjusted for the BMI of the investigated individuals and its translation to daily clinical practice needs to be viewed with caution if unadjusted values are showcased. Our results additionally revealed that the total nasal soft tissue thickness in the location of the DNA was related statistically significantly to gender, with men having greater thickness (*P* = .032), whereas BMI did not influence the thickness to this extent (*P* = .053) when calculating multifactorial models. This indicates that, independent of BMI, there is a statistically significant gender difference in the thickness of the nasal soft tissues, which again needs to be accounted for when interpreting data on nasal soft tissue anatomy.

The location of the artery was on average 2.6 ± 0.5 mm deep to the skin surface with a range of 1.7 to 3.8 mm indicating a variability of 2 mm within the investigated sample. Given the mean total soft tissue thickness of 4.45 ± 0.7 mm in this location, the artery can therefore be located in almost 50% of the total soft tissue extent, which highlights the risk of intra-arterial product application when targeting this area. When adjusting the depth of the artery to the total soft tissue thickness, it was found that, independent of gender, the artery is located at approximately 60% of the total soft tissue thickness with a range of 37.8% to 76.7%. This is remarkable because it confirms the suggestion to adjust values on nasal anatomy to gender and BMI to obtain data sets that facilitate generalizability to a larger population without having to stratify for gender or BMI. Clinically,

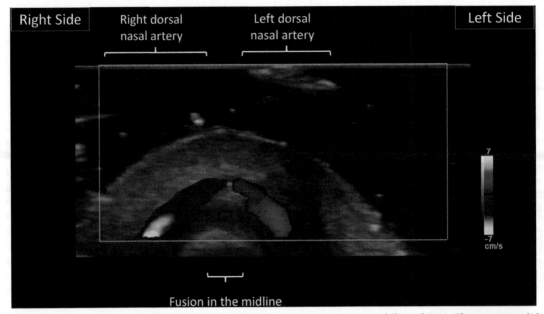

Fig. 3. Doppler-supported ultrasound image showing the anastomosis between bilateral DNA. The anastomosis is located in the subcutaneous layer superficial to the procerus muscle.

this results in an easier understanding and better applicability of presented results, which in turn increase patient safety when translated into daily practice.

The anastomosis of the DNA with the contralateral side in the midline of the nasal dorsum was on average 6.81 ± 3.0 mm inferior to the nasal radix for the entire study population (n = 51) with statistically significant difference between genders

(P = .009) as males have been shown to have a greater distance when compared with females. When correlating the distance measurements to the total length of the nose, no statistically significant relationship was identified. This is an interesting finding, which is explained by the vascular origin of the DNA. The DNA is one of the terminal branches of the ophthalmic artery and it is therefore connected to the intraorbital vascular

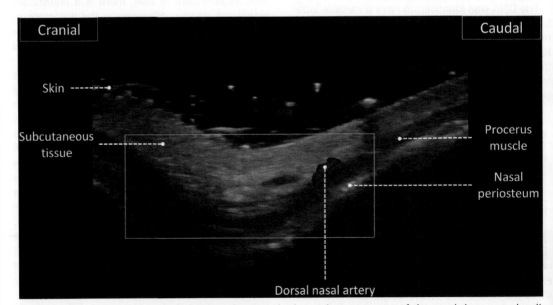

Fig. 4. Doppler-supported ultrasound image showing the layered arrangement of the nasal dorsum and radix. The DNA is located in the subcutaneous layer superficial to the procerus muscle.

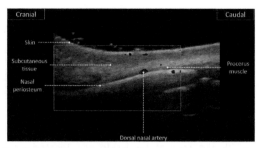

Fig. 5. Doppler-supported ultrasound image showing the layered arrangement of the nasal dorsum and radix. The DNA is located in the supraperiosteal layer deep to the procerus muscle.

network. It could be theorized that during development and growth of the individual the proximity to the ophthalmic artery is maintained despite the growth of the nose. Because this is just speculation without a scientific fundament, future studies elaborating the embryology of the facial vascular supply will be needed to reject or affirm the theory presented herein. It needs to be pointed out, that most minimally invasive corrections of the dorsal nose are performed in the cranial aspect of the nose that is in close proximity to the described location of the DNA. The authors want to emphasize that the close proximity of the DNA and the most frequently addressed area of the dorsum of the nose should be taken extremely serious by injectors and strengthens the recommendation that liquid rhinoplasties of the nose should only be performed by experienced injectors (**Fig. 6**).

The anatomy of the nasal radix is interesting because it contains the bony origin of the procerus muscle. This muscle has been shown by the applied ultrasound imaging to originate from the nasal bone and to become more superficial as it travels into the glabella to ultimately connect with the frontalis muscle. The DNA was found in 100% (n = 51) of the investigated cases to anastomose with the contralateral side in closest proximity to the bony origin of the muscle. Because the procerus muscle does not respect fascial layers along its course, the DNA can have two different positions in relation to the procerus muscle: superficial or deep to the muscle. Our results have revealed that the DNA was more frequently identified superficial to the procerus muscle (58.8%; n = 30) than deep to the muscle (41.2%; n = 21). Because the numbers are fairly similar, in practice, one should consider that the DNA can be observed in both locations and that this anatomic area is high risk because of the variable course of the DNA. Previous studies have suggested to inject in contact with bone, which is the most frequently performed technique based on the experience of the authors to avoid more superficially located arteries.[15,19] Because the DNA has an almost equal distribution of superficial and deep pathway in relation to the course of the procerus muscle previous findings need to be interpreted with caution. One potential reason why our results are not aligned with previous publications (8% vs 78%; deep vs superficial)[18] could be based on the sample investigated, because this study analyzed a White population and previous reports included Asian populations only. When stratifying the results by gender, it was observed that in women the DNA was located (n = 15; 62.5%) deep to the procerus muscle, whereas in men it was located (n = 21; 77.7%) superficial to the procerus muscle (P = .005). This underscores that results should not be presented and accepted on a general and unadjusted level because there is the potential that statistically significant differences exist depending on gender or body habitus. Previous studies have not conducted adjustments to the extent presented herein and therefore a critical re-evaluation of concepts is recommended.

In a previous literature review of 48 cases of blindness,[6] 56.3% (n = 27) followed nasal soft tissue filler injections. These unfortunate circumstances highlight the relevance of the results presented herein. Knowledge of nasal vascular anatomy is of the utmost importance to avoid severe adverse events with soft tissue filler injections. The results expand on previous studies and show that absolute and unadjusted values do not accurately reflect on the individual patient's anatomy. Moreover, adjustment for BMI and gender have revealed that there is a difference and understanding this can allow injectors to tailor treatments to safer outcomes. Previous studies have recommended to inject in contact with the bone[4,15,19] but our results have shown that the

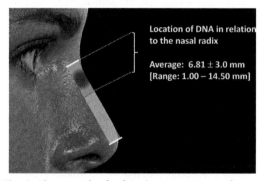

Fig. 6. Photograph of a female patient's nose from a lateral view depicting the vertical distribution of the dorsal nasal artery in relationship to the nasal radix. The *dark red area* represents the average location of the artery, and the *light red areas* represent the minimum and maximum range. In this study, no arteries coursed in the *green* area.

overall minimal distance between the DNA and the nasal periosteum is 0.90 mm. This highlights the high risk involved with injecting the nasal radix. These procedures should be performed with great care and by practitioners with intimate knowledge of the nasal anatomy. Although the number injectors across the world continues to grow, there are facial areas that are better suited for a novice injector; the nasal radix is not one of them.

This study also shows that the use of preinjection ultrasound might be of assistance when performing such high-risk procedures. Using preinjection ultrasound imaging allows the injector to visualize the targeted area and to identify the relationship to fascial layers and depth of the DNA. Observing the artery in close contact with the bone could suggest a more superficial injection, whereas identifying the artery in more superficial layers would dictate safer product placement in the supraperiosteal plane. In addition, this study has also shown in the investigated cohort that arterial vascular anatomy and especially the DNA has a highly variable course with almost equal distribution in coursing superficial or deep to the procerus muscle. This should be considered when injecting the nasal radix and incorporated into treatment algorithms and weighed with patient desire for aesthetic improvement.

SUMMARY

This ultrasound-based investigation was conducted in a large White sample (n = 51) and expanded on previous results obtained from Asian study populations. The results revealed that the DNA is highly variable in its course in relationship to the procerus muscle with approximately equal distribution of a superficial and deep pathway. Moreover, the underlying fascial and arterial anatomy is highly variable between genders and the depth of the artery is influenced by BMI. Adjusting the measurements showed that the DNA and its bilateral fusion is located at approximately 60% of the total soft tissue thickness and in an average distance of 6.8 mm inferior to the nasal radix. Understanding nasal layered and vascular anatomy can help to prevent serious adverse events if applied and interpreted appropriately.

CLINICS CARE POINTS

- Thorough knowledge about the topographical relationship of the arteries in the glabella region is crucial in order to avoid intra-

arterial injections of soft-tissue filler material which can ultimately result in permanent vision loss due to the occlusion of the ophthalmic artery.

- The dorsal nasal artery was identified to have a variable location in relationship to the procerus muscle: it can be located either superficial or deep to it.

- The anastomosis of the dorsal nasal artery with the contralateral side was located on average 6.81 mm inferior to the nasal radix.

DISCLOSURE

None of the authors listed have any commercial associations or financial disclosures that might pose or create a conflict of interest with the methods applied or the results presented in this article.

REFERENCES

1. Society TA. Aesthetic Plastic Surgery National Databank Statistics 2020. 2021. Available at: https://cdn.surgery.org/media/statistics/aestheticplasticsurgerynationaldatabank-2020stats.pdf. Accessed May 19, 2021.
2. Rho NK, Park JY, Youn CS, et al. Early changes in facial profile following structured filler rhinoplasty: an anthropometric analysis using a 3-dimensional imaging system. Dermatol Surg Off Publ Am Soc Dermatol Surg 2017;43(2):255–63.
3. Kassir R, Venkataram A, Malek A, et al. Non-surgical rhinoplasty: the ascending technique and a 14-year retrospective study of 2130 cases. Aesthetic Plast Surg 2020. https://doi.org/10.1007/s00266-020-02048-8.
4. Singh S. Practical tips and techniques for injection rhinoplasty. J Cutan Aesthet Surg 2019;12(1):60–2.
5. Rauso R, Colella G, Zerbinati N, et al. Safety and early satisfaction assessment of patients seeking nonsurgical rhinoplasty with filler. J Cutan Aesthet Surg 2017;10(4):207.
6. Beleznay K, Carruthers JDA, Humphrey S, et al. Update on avoiding and treating blindness from fillers: a recent review of the world literature. Aesthet Surg J 2019. https://doi.org/10.1093/asj/sjz053.
7. Cho K-HH, Dalla Pozza E, Toth G, et al. Pathophysiology study of filler-induced blindness. Aesthet Surg J 2019;39(1):96–106.
8. Michalinos A, Zogana S, Kotsiomitis E, et al. Anatomy of the ophthalmic artery: a review concerning its modern surgical and clinical applications. Anat Res Int 2015;2015:1–8.
9. Cotofana S, Lachman N. Arteries of the face and their relevance for minimally invasive facial

procedures: an anatomical review. Plast Reconstr Surg 2019;143(2):416–26.

10. Dey JK, Recker CA, Olson MD, et al. Assessing nasal soft-tissue envelope thickness for rhinoplasty: normative data and a predictive algorithm. JAMA Facial Plast Surg 2019;21(6):511–7.

11. Çavuş Özkan M, Yeşil F, Bayramiçli İ, et al. Soft tissue thickness variations of the nose: a radiological study. Aesthet Surg J 2020;40(7):711–8.

12. Pavicic T, Webb KL, Frank K, et al. Arterial wall penetration forces in needles versus cannulas. Plast Reconstr Surg 2019;143(3):504e–12e.

13. Rosengaus F, Nikolis A. Cannula versus needle in medical rhinoplasty: the nose knows. J Cosmet Dermatol 2020;19. https://doi.org/10.1111/jocd.13743.

14. Tansatit T, Moon H-J, Rungsawang C, et al. Safe planes for injection rhinoplasty: a histological analysis of midline longitudinal sections of the Asian nose. Aesthetic Plast Surg 2016;40(2):236–44.

15. Jung GS, Chu SG, Lee JW, et al. A safer non-surgical filler augmentation rhinoplasty based on the anatomy of the nose. Aesthetic Plast Surg 2019;43(2):447–52.

16. Moon H-J, Lee W, Do Kim H, et al. Doppler ultrasonographic anatomy of the midline nasal dorsum. Aesthetic Plast Surg 2020. https://doi.org/10.1007/s00266-020-02025-1.

17. Choi DY, Bae JH, Youn KH, et al. Topography of the dorsal nasal artery and its clinical implications for augmentation of the dorsum of the nose. J Cosmet Dermatol 2018;17(4):637–42.

18. Lee W, Kim J-S, Oh W, et al. Nasal dorsum augmentation using soft tissue filler injection. J Cosmet Dermatol 2019;18. https://doi.org/10.1111/jocd.13018.

19. Chen B, Ma L, Ji K, et al. Rhinoplasty with hyaluronic acid: a standard 5-step injection procedure using sharp needle. Ann Plast Surg 2020;85(6). Available at: https://journals.lww.com/annalsplasticsurgery/Fulltext/2020/12000/Rhinoplasty_With_Hyaluronic_Acid__A_Standard.5.aspx.

The Columellar Arteries in the Asian Nose

Benrita Jitaree, PhD[a], Thirawass Phumyoo, PhD[b],*

KEYWORDS

- Columellar artery • Artery of nose • Columella • Nasal tip • Rhinoplasty • Filler injection

KEY POINTS

- The columellar artery courses within the columella from deep to superficial along with the columellar base to the nasal tip.
- For increasing nasal tip projection, filler is recommended to inject into the deep fatty layer between the medial crus of lower lateral cartilage and the supraperiosteal layer at the anterior nasal spine in the midline to avoid the vascular compromise.
- For operative rhinoplasty at the columella, the meticulous dissection should be performed adherent to the perichondrium of lower lateral cartilage, and subdermal defatting of nasal tip skin should be avoided due to numerous arterial plexuses in the superficial plane.

INTRODUCTION

The nose serves a considerable aesthetic role creating the balance at the center of face. The morphologic characteristics of Asian nose are a short or retracted columella, an acute nasolabial angle, deficient tip projection, and frail underlying cartilaginous segments.[1] Asian tend to obtain thicker skin and an ample subcutaneous tissue at the nasolabial angle than Caucasians to minimize the undulating appearance. Thus, the aesthetic procedures have increased dramatically worldwide to contour the facial shape and correct several aging characteristics.[2]

Nowadays, both surgical rhinoplasty and filler rhinoplasty are considered the most popular aesthetic approach to improve the columellar angle and a tip of the nose in Asia.[3,4] Due to the dissimilarities of aesthetic criteria among different populations, it is not easy to indicate an ideal angle for the most appealing columella. Nevertheless, a range of 90° to 110° of the nasolabial angle might help for an individual attractive look.[1,5]

During a rhinoplasty approach, improper intervention, either by transcolumellar incision or filler injection at the columellar base and membranous septum, can lead to severing of the arterial distribution in the columella.[3,4] Complications as skin necrosis and deformity may arise from inadequate blood supply to the columella following aesthetic interventions.[3,4] Consequently, it is necessary to perform the ideal aesthetic approach by understanding the detailed configurations of the columellar artery (CoA) that might help the physician to minimize the chances of adverse events. This article aims at a comprehensive review of the CoA in Asians who have different nasal features from the other ethnicity. Moreover, the clinical aspects associated with Asian CoA are further concluded for giving the knowledge to assist the clinician during performing the nasal aesthetic procedure.

Five layers of the nasal columella

- Skin: Generally, nasal skin varies significantly with the proportions of fibrous tissue and sebaceous glands in different portions of the nose, and columellar skin is thinner and less sebaceous than the skin at the dorsum of nose. The external part of columellar skin is

[a] Chakri Naruebodindra Medical Institute, Faculty of Medicine Ramathibodi Hospital, Mahidol University, 270 Rama VI Road, Ratchatewi, Bangkok 10400, Thailand; [b] Department of Basic Medical Science, Faculty of Medicine Vajira Hospital, Navamindradhiraj University, Bangkok 10300, Thailand
* Corresponding author.
E-mail address: oncestep@hotmail.com

Facial Plast Surg Clin N Am 30 (2022) 143–148
https://doi.org/10.1016/j.fsc.2022.01.014

tightly attached to the medial crura and connected with vestibular skin internally.[3]

- Superficial fatty layer: At the columellar septum, adipose tissue that is loosely attached to the overlying skin with oriented fibrous septae and traveling subdermal vascular network can be found. Rostrally, the fat pad at the supratip is densely connected to dermis, and the interdermal fat pad is located caudally from the supratip fat between both, the medial and middle crus.[3]
- Fibromuscular layer: The depressor septi nasi muscle is located between the superficial and deep fatty layers deep within the lip near the columellar base. It originated from the incisive fossa of the maxilla and inserts into the mobile portion of the nasal septum and intermingles with the deep muscle fibers of the orbicularis oris muscle. This muscle acts for pulling down the tip of the nose to enlarge the nostrils.[1,3,5]
- Deep fatty layer: A deep loose areolar tissue layer underneath the fibromuscular layer that lacks fibrous septa.[3]
- Perichondrium: A longitudinal fibrous sheath under the deep fatty layer covered the septal cartilage.[3]

Vascular supply of the columella

Unfortunately, previous literature reviews have indicated that few studies investigated the vascular network at the nasal tip and columella in Asians. The artery at the columella is formed by many arterial branches of both external carotid and internal carotid arteries, for example, the septal branches of superior labial artery (SLA), the inferior alar, and lateral nasal branches of facial artery, and the dorsal nasal branch of ophthalmic artery.

Blood supply sources below the level of columellar base (**Figs. 1–3**).

There are the tributaries of the facial artery at the superior labial region and the nasal base which arises from the external carotid system.[6–9] The SLA bifurcates from the facial artery in the vicinity of oral commissure to travel along the vermillion of upper lip in the layer between the orbicularis oris muscle and the oral mucosa with the depth from mucosa of 3 to 4 mm.[6,7,10] In some cases, the SLA locates superficial to the muscular layer to anastomose with the superficial septal branches of the nose. The SLA situates about 9 mm superior to the vermillion border of upper lip and descends below the border about 5 to 6 mm at the midline.[6] The diameter of SLA ranges from 0.3 to 3.0 mm.[6,10] Commonly, the arteries of both sides

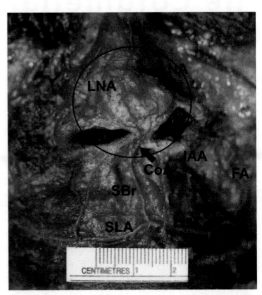

Fig. 1. Cadaveric dissection reveals many sources of vessels that supply the columella: AA, angular artery; DNA, dorsal nasal artery; LNA, lateral nasal artery; CoA, columellar artery; IAA, inferior alar artery; SBr, septal branch of superior labial artery; SLA, superior labial artery; FA, facial artery.

have a midline anastomosis, while a unilateral absence is very rare. The SLA ramifies the ascending vertical branches as the superficial and deep septal branches in the philtrum toward the nasal septum.[6,10] The deep septal branch is situated underneath the orbicularis muscle, and the superficial septal branch proceeds cranially on the muscle. The external diameters range from 0.3 to 1.1 mm for the deep septal branch and range from 0.4 to 1.5 mm for the superficial septal branch.[6] Both septal branches travel across the columellolabial junction and continue as the CoA in 72.5%.[5] Furthermore, at the base of ala, the facial artery ramifies occasionally a short trunk to give off the inferior alar artery (IAA) which proceeds directly toward the ala.[6] This trunk was founded in 53% to 57% of cases with the external diameter less than 1 mm. The IAA is running along the nasal base to anastomose with the CoA at the midline in 27.5%.

Blood supply sources above the level of nasal tip

Rostral to the columella, the CoA anastomoses with the tributaries of both the external carotid and the internal carotid systems via the lateral nasal branch of facial artery from the ala of nose and the dorsal nasal branch of ophthalmic artery from the dorsum of nose, respectively (see **Figs. 1–3**).[5] At the base of nose level, the lateral nasal

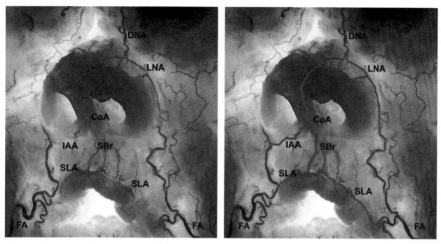

Fig. 2. Translucent image underwent modified Sihler staining procedure that exposes the arterial anastomosis of columellar artery (lateral view of left side): DNA, dorsal nasal artery; LNA, lateral nasal artery; CoA, columellar artery; IAA, inferior alar artery; SBr, septal branch of superior labial artery; SLA, superior labial artery; FA, facial artery.

artery (LNA) ramifies from either a short trunk with the IAA or the independent main trunk of facial artery.[6] It proceeds along the alar-facial crease above the fibromuscular layer with the distance superior to the alar groove of about 4 mm and the external diameter of approximately 1.5 mm. Then, it bends inwardly in an arc shape distributing across the nasal tip to anastomose with the CoA.

The dorsal nasal artery (DNA) emerges from the ophthalmic artery close to the medial orbital rim about 8 to 13 mm above the medial canthal tendon.[11] The DNA is not a constant artery

because it might originate as either the bilateral DNA or the unilateral DNA.[11,12] When the DNA appears as unilateral, it often presents with a large arterial diameter. The artery travels in the superficial fatty layer to enter the radix zone and descends downward on the dorsum of nose with a larger diameter.[11–13] The DNA is located on average at 4.4 mm, 4.6 mm, and 5.2 mm lateral to the midline of the nose on the intercanthal, quadrisected, and bisected lines, respectively.[12] At the cartilaginous portion of nose, it courses more deeply under the fibromuscular layer and communicates with the LNA and the CoA. Tiny

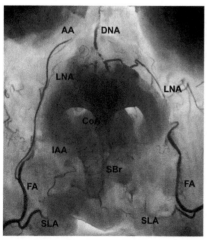
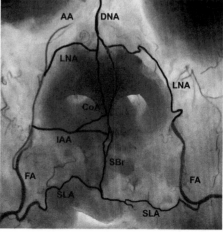

Fig. 3. Translucent image underwent modified Sihler staining procedure that exposes the arterial anastomosis of columellar artery (anterior view): AA, angular artery; DNA, dorsal nasal artery; LNA, lateral nasal artery; CoA, columellar artery; IAA, inferior alar artery; SBr, septal branch of superior labial artery; SLA, superior labial artery; FA, facial artery.

arterial branches from the septal artery and the IAA form the vascular plexus at the base of nose, whereas the LNA and DNA establish the vascular plexus in the tip of nose.[5,11]

Columellar artery

The nasal cartilage of the columella consists of 3 pieces of cartilage including 1 septal cartilage in the midline and 2 medial cruses of lower lateral cartilage at each side of the nasal tip (see **Figs. 1–3**).[3] The CoA courses anteriorly in the columella toward the nasal tip and inferior to the medial crus of lower lateral cartilage, and then forms the arterial plexus with the arterial branches from the nasal dorsum.[1,5] This artery could be classified into 4 types depending on the number of arteries at the columella: *type 1* – one CoA in 50% (**Fig. 4**), *type 2* – double CoA in 37.3% (**Fig. 5**), *type 3* – forked type of CoA in 7.8%, and *type 4* – Absent of CoA in 3.9%. The external diameters range from 0.2 to 0.33 mm.[5] At the base of septum, the CoA travels deeply closer to the medial crus with the depth from skin of 1.5 to 2.5 mm, whereas at the nasal infratip, the CoA runs evenly between the medial crus and the epidermis in the deep fatty layer.[1] Nevertheless, the CoA and other small vessels are absent on the deep plane at the anterior nasal spine.

Clinical relevance

Previous studies have revealed that common filler injection sites are nose, glabella, and forehead; 33.55%, 21.35%, and 18.3%, respectively.[14,15] The CoA is correlated with the nasal filler injection in Asian people. The first purpose of this approach is an improvement of the nasofrontal angle which is the angle between the nasal dorsum and the caudal forehead. In ideal Asian face, this angle should be range between 125° and 135°. Secondly, the straight nose and nasal tip projection should be taller than the projection of the nasal dorsum with a nasolabial angle ranging between 90° and 110°. An injection at the nasal dorsum might cause an intravascular occlusion of the DNA and the LNA because both vessels are located on the dorsum of nose, whereas the CoA might be injected during columellar injection.

The columellar injection, corresponding with nasal spine filler injection, is beneficial for nasal tip elevation and improves the nasolabial angle.[16] To increase the nasal tip projection, an injection is preferred to operate in the deep fatty layer, the injection site between the medial crus of lower lateral cartilage and the supraperiosteal layer at the anterior nasal spine. The advantage of injection in this plane is the reduction of the risk of injection into or damaging the vessels due to the lack of blood vessels.[2,17] A 23-G blunt cannula is highly recommended because it is larger than the diameter of the CoA. Thus, the chance of intravascular injection is lower than the small cannula. Both retrograde and linear threading techniques are generally suggested in the midline to prevent nasal tip deviation.[2] The volume of injection should range at 0.2 cc for the nasal columella and 0.5 cc for the anterior nasal spine. Aspiration is globally endorsed for confirming vascular injection. After injection, capillary refill should immediately be investigated for examining nasal blood supply.[18] According to the nasal tip injection area, the entire areas are predominantly associated with the CoA.

Although surgical rhinoplasty is one of the most popular aesthetic surgeries in Asian, risks are comparably similar in terms of vascular damage. Likely, the CoA might be damaged during the creation of the nasal tip projection by transcolumellar

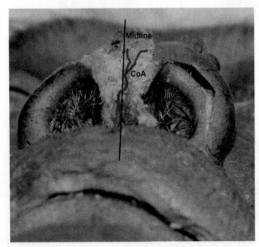

Fig. 4. Type 1 of the columellar artery is found with single arterial branch in 50% of cases; CoA, columellar artery.

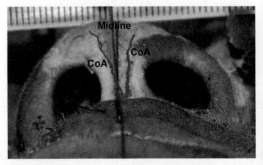

Fig. 5. Type 2 of the columellar artery which is found with double arterial branch in 37.3% of cases; CoA, columellar artery.

incision. In this case, the collateral circulation is of uttermost importance for the vascular supply and consecutively for the healing of the columella, as the main blood supply is lost.[19] The LNA from the facial artery and the DNA from the ophthalmic artery contribute to the vascular supply of the columella. In case of columellar reconstruction, the LNA within the nasolabial fold tissue pedicle is commonly used.[19] Meticulous surgical technique must be used when exposing the distal nasal framework. The plane of dissection should adhere to the perichondrium of lower lateral cartilage. In addition, the dissection should not proceed superiorly into the soft-tissue plane above the alar groove and subdermal defatting of nasal tip skin should be also kept away to avoid the superficial vascular plexus from the LNA and the DNA.

Prevalence of complications

Nasal filler augmentation is an alternative option for Asians who are worried about the potential complications of surgical rhinoplasty. However, numerous studies reported severe complications following nasal filler augmentations. An iatrogenic intravascular injection is indicated as the cause of disastrous complications including vascular compromise, skin necrosis, and blindness.[4,20] The visual loss after nasal filler injection was reported in most cases with 40.9% of the cases who is obtained the single nasal filler injection.[21] Moreover, blindness cases from Korea, China, and Thailand were 36.4%, 25%, and 6.8%, respectively. This complication was also found in Taiwan and USA; 4.5% and 2.3%.[21]

DISCUSSION

According to the anatomic data and the clinical correlation, the CoA should be recognized when the clinician decide to increase the nasal tip projection by injecting the columella and anterior nasal spine. Compared with the nasal dorsum injection, the injection of the columellar is less likely to cause vision loss as the CoA is supplied mainly by arterial branches which are located below the columellar base including the septal branches of SLA and the IAA. However, there is arterial anastomosis between the CoA and the DNA at the nasal tip which is a possible pathway of the filler from the columella to the ophthalmic artery.[1,5,11–13] An iatrogenic intravascular injection with high pressure could push the filler retrograde along the DNA and the ophthalmic artery, and then occludes the central retinal artery resulting in visual impairment (see **Fig. 1**).

Direct intravascular injection, external vascular compression, vascular injury, and vasospasm are the causes of vascular compromises. For the intravascular injection, the filler can move along the course of vessels and obstruct the vascular lumen. In terms of external compression, the injected filler is placed near the vessel and produces high pressure surrounding the vessel, which can then lead to the obstruction of the arterial circulation.[22] Nevertheless, the vascular compromise which can be found in the reported case of nasal tip augmentation is caused by the vascular compression of filler. Because of the limited tissue space of the nasal tip and nasal columella, the injected filler might compress the vessels.[16] Intravascular injection after nasal tip procedures is rare as the CoA has a smaller arterial diameter than most needles or cannulas. Previous studies showed that the range of the diameter of the CoA was approximately between 0.2 and 0.33 mm compared with the 29 G cannula (0.343 mm). The recommended cannula should not be smaller than 29 G.[18] Although the chance of intraarterial injection is rare, needle aspiration and checking of capillary refill are still strongly advised.

Most cases of vision loss after nasal augmentation can be explained by retrograde flow which can be caused by an intravascular injection pressure that is higher than the systolic arterial pressure. Then, the filler moves retrogradely along the vessel until reaching the proximal area to the origin of the central retinal artery. On the release of injection pressure, the arterial systemic blood pressure can move the filler into the ophthalmic artery and its branches, so the blood flow is blocked by filler leading to create symptoms such as blur vision or a vision loss.[23] Although the injection is conducted in the area which is not supplied by branches of the ophthalmic artery, the arterial communicating pathway between internal and external carotid arteries may bring the filler to the ophthalmic artery. The severe complications are discovered not only in vision loss but also skin necrosis which is ischemia of nasal tissue caused by arterial lumen blockage. In such complication cases, hyaluronidase may be a key to correction of the complication.[24]

SUMMARY

This article reviews the comprehensive information of the CoA in Asians who have different nasal features than other ethnicities. To decrease the risk of complications, a physician should deeply understand the nasal vascular anatomy such as vascular location, depth, and variation. In addition, the relationship between vessels and the other important facial tissue structures and the facial layers is crucial for the clinician.

CLINICS CARE POINTS

- The nose serves a considerable aesthetic role creating the balance at the center of face.
- Physicians should deeply understand the nasal vascular anatomy such as vascular location, depth, and variation.
- The nasal columella consists of five layers.
- The arteries at the columella are formed by many arterial branches of both external carotid and internal carotid arteries.

DISCLOSURE

The authors have nothing to disclose.

REFERENCES

1. Lee YI, Yang HM, Pyeon HJ, et al. Anatomical and histological study of the arterial distribution in the columellar area, and the clinical implications. Surg Radiol Anat 2014;36(7):669–74.
2. Moon HJ, Gao ZW, Hu ZQ, et al. Expert Consensus on Hyaluronic Acid Filler Facial Injection for Chinese Patients. Plast Reconstr Surg Glob Open 2020; 8(10):e3219.
3. Kim TK, Jeong JY. Surgical anatomy for Asian rhinoplasty. Arch Craniofac Surg 2019;20(3):147–57.
4. Moon HJ. Injection Rhinoplasty Using Filler. Facial Plast Surg Clin North Am 2018;26(3):323–30.
5. Jung DH, Kim HJ, Koh KS, et al. Arterial supply of the nasal tip in Asians. Laryngoscope 2000;110(2 Pt 1):308–11.
6. Lee HJ, Won SY, O J., et al. The facial artery: A Comprehensive Anatomical Review. Clin Anat 2018;31(1):99–108.
7. Phumyoo T, Tansatit T, Rachkeaw N. The soft tissue landmarks to avoid injury to the facial artery during filler and neurotoxin injection at the nasolabial region. J Craniofac Surg 2014;25(5):1885–9.
8. Jitaree B, Phumyoo T, Uruwan S, et al. Clinical implications of the arterial supplies and their anastomotic territories in the nasolabial region for avoiding arterial complications during soft tissue filler injection. Clin Anat 2021;34(4):581–9.
9. Tansatit T, Kenny E, Phumyoo T, et al. Cadaveric Dissections to Determine Surface Landmarks Locating the Facial Artery for Filler Injections. Aesthet Surg J 2021;41(6):NP550–8.
10. Tansatit T, Apinuntrum P, Phetudom T. A typical pattern of the labial arteries with implication for lip augmentation with injectable fillers. Aesthet Plast Surg 2014;38(6):1083–9.
11. Tansatit T, Apinuntrum P, Phetudom T. Facing the Worst Risk: Confronting the Dorsal Nasal Artery, Implication for Non-surgical Procedures of Nasal Augmentation. Aesthet Plast Surg 2017;41(1):191–8.
12. Choi DY, Bae JH, Youn KH, et al. Topography of the dorsal nasal artery and its clinical implications for augmentation of the dorsum of the nose. J Cosmet Dermatol 2018;17(4):637–42.
13. Tansatit T, Moon HJ, Rungsawang C, et al. Safe Planes for Injection Rhinoplasty: A Histological Analysis of Midline Longitudinal Sections of the Asian Nose. Aesthet Plast Surg 2016;40(2):236–44.
14. Sorensen EP, Council ML. Update in Soft-Tissue Filler-Associated Blindness. Dermatol Surg 2020; 46(5):671–7.
15. Jung GS. Clinical Aesthetics of the Nose for Filler Injection. Facial Plast Surg 2019;35(5):561–2.
16. Liew S, Scamp T, de Maio M, et al. Efficacy and Safety of a Hyaluronic Acid Filler to Correct Aesthetically Detracting or Deficient Features of the Asian Nose: A Prospective, Open-Label, Long-Term Study. Aesthet Surg J 2016;36(7):760–72.
17. Youn SH, Seo KK. Filler Rhinoplasty Evaluated by Anthropometric Analysis. Dermatol Surg 2016; 42(9):1071–81.
18. Tanaka Y, Matsuo K, Yuzuriha S. Westernization of the asian nose by augmentation of the retropositioned anterior nasal spine with an injectable filler. Eplasty 2011;11:e7.
19. Yang TH, Hsu NJ, Li CN. Both the Filler Amount and Columellar Elasticity Are Important in Injection Rhinoplasty in the Columella. Dermatol Surg 2019; 45(10):1339–42.
20. Nguyen JD, Duong H. Anatomy, Head and Neck, Lateral Nasal Artery. In: StatPearls. Treasure Island. FL; 2022.
21. Kapoor KM, Kapoor P, Heydenrych I, et al. Vision Loss Associated with Hyaluronic Acid Fillers: A Systematic Review of Literature. Aesthet Plast Surg 2020;44(3):929–44.
22. Weinberg MJ, Solish N. Complications of hyaluronic acid fillers. Facial Plast Surg 2009;25(5):324–8.
23. Lazzeri D, Agostini T, Figus M, et al. Blindness following cosmetic injections of the face. Plast Reconstr Surg 2012;129(4):995–1012.
24. Wibowo A, Kapoor KM, Philipp-Dormston WG. Reversal of Post-filler Vision Loss and Skin Ischaemia with High-Dose Pulsed Hyaluronidase Injections. Aesthet Plast Surg 2019;43(5):1337–44.

3D Anthropometric Facial Imaging - A comparison of different 3D scanners

Konstantin Christoph Koban, MD[a,*], Philipp Perko, MD[a], Zhouxiao Li, MD[a], Ya Xu, MD[a], Riccardo E. Giunta, MD, PhD[a], Michael G. Alfertshofer[a], Lukas H. Kohler, MD[a], David L. Freytag, MD[b], Sebastian Cotofana, MD, PhD[c], Konstantin Frank, MD[a]

KEYWORDS

• 3D scan • Three-dimensional surface imaging • Anthropometry • Facial imaging

INTRODUCTION

Three-dimensional (3D) imaging has been proved to be a valuable tool in the preoperative, intraoperative, and postoperative setting for facial plastic surgeons and dermatologists.[1–12] Accurate depiction of the face has become a helpful adjunct in the preoperative setting during patient consultation and operative planning.[7,10,13,14] 3D imaging has, furthermore, shown to be of great use in the intraoperative setting to assess for changes of symmetry and provide objective feedback to the surgeon on the way to the desired surgical outcome.[12,15] Moreover, 3D is on its way to be the gold standard for postoperative assessment of volume- and shape-altering surgeries and minimally invasive interventions, not only in the hospital and private practice setting but also in the field of research. A plethora of studies have shown that 3D imaging allows to assess postinterventional changes in a meticulous manner and enables the transition from subjective outcome assessment to objective outcome assessment, strengthening the efforts to move minimally invasive treatments from an eminence- to an evidence-based endeavor.[2,3,7,13,16–19] 3D imaging devices have evolved from complex stationary systems to portable systems, which can be used in a multitude of situations and locations.[5,10,12] However, especially in facial plastic surgery measurement deviations can be misguiding the surgeon and become rather a hazard than a supporting tool. A measurement deviation of 3 mm might be considered as acceptable in breast surgery; however, a difference of 3 mm can cause a nose to look harmonious or unharmonious.

It is thus essential to investigate the measurement deviations when scanning with different 3D imaging systems. Thus, the objective of this investigation was to evaluate the accuracy and reliability of standard 3D anthropometric measurements of the face made with one low-cost handheld 3D scanner and one industrial-type mobile 3D scanner.

MATERIALS AND METHODS
Subjects

A total of 30 healthy volunteers (15 males and 15 females) were enrolled into this study. Mean age of the participants was 32.0 ± 9.0 years with a mean body mass index of 26.1 ± 5.0 kg/m^2. All volunteers were screened for exclusionary criteria, including a history of either unilateral or bilateral facial procedures/surgery, trauma, or diseases that could alter facial anatomy. This study was

Funding: This study received no funding.
[a] Division of Hand, Plastic and Aesthetic Surgery, University Hospital, LMU Munich, Munich, Germany;
[b] Department of Plastic Surgery, Community Hospital Havelhöhe, Berlin; [c] Department of Clinical Anatomy, Mayo Clinic College of Medicine and Science, Rochester, MN, USA
* Corresponding author. Division of Hand, Plastic and Aesthetic Surgery, University Hospital, LMU Munich, Pettenkoferstraße 8a, 80336 Munich, Germany.
E-mail address: Konstantin.koban@med.uni-muenchen.de

Facial Plast Surg Clin N Am 30 (2022) 149–158
https://doi.org/10.1016/j.fsc.2022.01.003
1064-7406/22/

Table 1
Table showing the 17 landmarks used to reconstruct the consecutively performed distance measurements

Abbreviation/Full Name	Definition
Trichinion	Trichion, widow's peak
G (glabella)	Bulge between the 2 eyebrows and the most prominent point on the median sagittal plane
N (nasion)	Intersection point of the frontal bone and 2 nasal bones of the human skull
Pronasale	Nasal apex
C'c (columella center)	Midpoint of the columella crest at the level of the nostril top points
Sn (subnasale center)	Columellar base
Ls	Midpoint of the upper vermilion line
Sto (stomion)	Midpoint of closed lip
Li	Midpoint of the lower vermilion line
Sl (sublabiale)	Most posterior midpoint on the labiomental soft tissue contour
Gn (gnathion)	Lowest point of the mandible in the median sagittal plane
Endocanthion	Endocanthion bilateral
Exocanthion	Exocanthion bilateral
Al (alar lateral)	Most lateral point on alar contour bilateral
C' (columella)	Columella bilateral
Septum nasale	Point at each margin of the midportion of the columella crest
Ch (cheilion)	Oral commissure bilateral

Landmark positions were defined according to Farkas and colleagues[26] and Swennen and colleagues.[27]

performed in adherence with the Declaration of Helsinki (1996)[20] and was previously approved by the Ethics Committee of the Ludwig-Maximilian University, Munich, Germany, under the number (Reference Number 266-13). Written informed consent was obtained from all participants for the use of their facial images and personal data for research purposes and publication before inclusion in the study.

3D Imaging

Subjects removed any jewelry and hair from the face, forehead, and ears to give full exposure of the area to be scanned. Male volunteers were asked to shave. All volunteers were asked to close their mouth without clenching the teeth and had to remain in a relaxed, neutral facial expression on the same chair with a fixed backrest. Volunteers had to take an upright, nonexcessive sitting position and close their eyes. Light conditions and background were not specifically changed in our consultation room to achieve conditions similar to real-life application. 3D Scan imaging was performed for each session with the mobile Sense 3D Scanner (3D Systems, South Carolina. USA), mobile Artec Eva (Artec 3D, Luxembourg) scanner, and the Vectra XT 3D Surface Imaging System (Canfield Inc, NJ, USA).

Conducted Measurements

A total of 17 anatomic landmarks were defined using the Mirror application (Canfield Scientific; NJ, USA). A total of 37 measurements were performed between those landmarks. The specified anatomic landmarks and the respective distance measurements are given in **Tables 1** and **2**. In addition, the upper face to face height index, lower face to face index, and mandibula to upper face height index were calculated using the Mirror application software.

Statistical Analysis

Analyses were performed using SPSS Statistics 27 (IBM, Armonk, NY, USA). The data are shown as the means ± standard deviations, numbers, or percentages. Levene test was used to evaluate the distribution of quantitative data, and paired t test was used for data comparisons between the reference system (Vectra XT) and both mobile scanners (Sense and Artec). Differences were considered statistically significant at a probability level of 0.05 or less to guide conclusions.

RESULTS
Distance Measurements

Comparing all direct landmark measurements derived from the reference system, a mean

Table 2
Table displaying the respective investigated distances

Abbreviation/Full Name	Definition
Upper face-face height index	Nasion-stomion/ nasion-gnathion
Lower face-face height index	Subnasale-gnathion/ nasion-gnathion
Mandibula-face height index	Stomion-gnathion/ nasion-gnathion
Mandibula-upper face height index	Stomion-gnathion/ nasion-stomion
Mandibula-lower face height index	Stomion-gnathion/ subnasale-gnathion
Nasal index	Alare(r)-alare(l)/ nasion-subnasale
Upper lip height-mouth width index	Subnasale-stomion/ chelion(r)-chelion(l)
Cutaneous-total upper lip height index	Subnasale-labiale superius/ subnasale-stomion
Vermilion-total upper lip height index	Labiale superius-Stomion/ Subnasale-Stomion
Vermilion-cutaneous upper lip height index	Labiale superius-stomion/ subnasale-labiale superius
Vermilion height index	Labiale superius-stomion/stomion-labiale inferius
Intercanthal-nasal width index	Endocanthion(r)-endocanthion(l)/ alare(r)-alare(l)
Nose-face height index	Nasion-subnasale/ nasion-gnathion
Nose-mouth width index	Alare(r)-alare(l)/ chelion(r)-chelion(l)
Upper lip-upper face height index	Subnasale-stomion/ nasion-stomion
Upper lip-mandible height index	Subnasale-stomion/ stomion-gnathion
Lower lip-face height index	Stomion-sublabiale/ subnasale-gnathion
Lower lip-mandible height index	Stomion-sublabiale/ stomion-gnathion
Nose-face height index	Nasion-subnasale/ nasion-gnathion

(continued on next page)

Table 2
(continued)

Abbreviation/Full Name	Definition
Nose-mouth width index	Alare(r)-alare(l)/ chelion(r)-chelion(l)
Upper lip-upper face height index	Subnasale-stomion/ nasion-stomion
Upper lip-mandible height index	Subnasale-stomion/ stomion-gnathion
Lower lip-face height index	Stomion-sublabiale/ subnasale-gnathion
Lower lip-mandible height index	Stomion-sublabiale/ stomion-gnathion
Nasal tip protrusion width index	Subnasale-pronasale/ alare(r)-alare(l)
Nasal tip protrusion-nose height index	Subnasale-pronasale/ nasion-subnasale
Lower-upper lip height index	Stomion-sublabiale/ subnasale-stomion
Cutaneous lower-upper lip height index	Labiale inferius-sublabiale/ subnasale-labiale superius
Vermilion-total lower lip height index	Stomion-labiale inferius/stomion-sublabiale
Vermilion-cutaneous lower lip height index	Stomion-labiale inferius/labiale inferius-sublabiale
Cutaneous-total lower lip height index	Labiale inferius-sublabiale/ stomion-sublabiale
Intercanthal-mouth width index	Endocanthion(r)-endocanthion(l)/ chelion(r)-chelion(l)
Nose-upper face height index	Nasion-subnasale/ nasion-stomion
Nasal bridge index	Nasion-pronasale/ nasion-subnasale
Interalar width	Distance between Al(r) to Al(l)
Columella length	Distance between Sn to c'(c)
Nasofrontal angle	Angle from G to N to Ntp

l: left; r:right; Al: Ala; G:Glabella; N:Nasion; Ntp: Nasal tip; Sn: Subnasale; c'(c): columella center

deviation of 0.13 ± 2.71 mm (range: -10.26 to 13.9 mm) was found with the Artec scanner and -0.19 ± 3.8 mm (range: -14.09 to 18.9 mm) with the Sense scanner.

Table 3
Table displaying the respective measured distances for the facial measurements with the Vectra 3D imaging system (reference) and the Artec and the Sense 3D mobile scanners (±1 standard deviation) and the respective P values

Abbreviation/Full Name	Vectra	Artec	P Value	Sense	P Value
Widow's peak-nasion	65.77 (9.2)	66.31 (8.5)	.454	67.23 (7.8)	.251
Exocanthion(r)-exocanthion(l)	94.23 (4.5)	95.62 (4.2)	.017[a]	100.99 (6.8)	< .001[b]
Endocanthion(r)-endocanthion(l)	27.87 (2.0)	28.42 (2.6)	.168	29.25 (2.6)	.009[a]
Nasion-subnasale	56.66 (3.9)	56.54 (3.6)	.837	57.04 (2.5)	.595
Subnasale-pronasale	19.48 (1.4)	19.82 (1.9)	.330	19.41 (2.0)	.872
Subnasale-stomion	22.41 (2.9)	21.55 (2.5)	.016[a]	20.57 (2.6)	< .001[b]
Stomion-sublabiale	17.86 (2.3)	17.54 (2.0)	.341	17.84 (1.8)	.967
Nasion-stomion	77.75 (3.7)	77.04 (3.3)	.222	76.04 (3.4)	.006[a]
Nasion-gnathion	120.84 (6.5)	120.33 (5.2)	.527	118.93 (5.1)	.043[a]
Alare(r)-alare(l)	30.23 (3.0)	31.08 (3.5)	.004[a]	28.49 (3.8)	< .001[b]
Columella apex(c)-subnasale	9.76 (2.1)	10.98 (2.4)	< .001[a]	10.18 (2.2)	.388
Subnasale-gnathion	66.15 (5.0)	66.59 (4.8)	.438	64.53 (4.8)	.035[a]
Stomion-gnathion	43.79 (4.0)	44.92 (3.0)	.058	44.71 (3.4)	.135
Chelion(r)-chelion(l)	53.56 (3.9)	50.94 (3.9)	< .001[b]	51.14 (4.8)	< .001[b]
Subnasale-labiale superius	14.57 (2.8)	13.67 (2.3)	.038[a]	13.69 (2.3)	.075
Labiale superius-stomion	8.49 (1.6)	8.76 (1.8)	.365	7.32 (1.1)	< .001[b]
Labiale inferius-stomion	7.69 (2.0)	7.63 (2.1)	.802	8.20 (1.7)	.117
Labiale inferius-sublabiale	11.37 (1.3)	11.51 (1.6)	.627	10.44 (2.1)	.004[a]
Sublabiale-gnathion	26.81 (2.4)	27.57 (2.5)	.122	26.98 (2.7)	.730

[a] $P < .05$
[b] $P < .001$

Measurements for the distances obtained with the investigated scanners are shown in **Table 3** with their respective averaged values and standard deviation, as well as P values when testing for statistically significant differences.

Facial Measurements

Facial indices for the observed scanners are shown in **Table 4** with their respective averaged values and 1 standard deviation, as well as statistical difference to the reference measurement (Vectra) as P value. The Artec and Sense mobile scanners measured statistically significant different values for the mandibula-face height index with $P = .0012$ and $P = .004$, respectively; for the mandibula-upper face height index with $P = .022$ and $P < .001$, respectively; and for the mandibula-lower face height index with $P = .021$ and $P < .001$, respectively (see **Table 4**).

NASAL MEASUREMENTS

Nasal measurements for the observed scanners are shown in **Tables 5 and 6** with their respective

averaged values and 1 standard deviation, as well as statistical difference to the reference measurement (Vectra) as P value. The Artec measured the nasal index, nose-mouth width index, interalar width, and the columella length statistically different with $P = .017$, $P < .001$, $P = .038$, and $P < .001$, respectively, when compared with the Vectra. The Sense measured the nasal index, intercanthal-nasal width index, the nose-upper face height index, nasal bridge index, interalar width, nasofrontal angle, and nasal tip protrusion width index statistically different with $P = .002$, $P < .001$, $P = .013$, $P = .013$, $P < .001$, and $P = .008$, respectively, when compared with the Vectra.

PERIORAL MEASUREMENTS

Perioral measurements for the observed scanners are shown in **Table 5** with their respective averaged values and 1 standard deviation, as well as statistical difference to the reference measurement (Vectra) as P value. The Artec measured the upper lip-mandible height index and the intercanthal-mouth width index statistically

Table 4
Table showing the mean measured indices (±1 standard deviation) for the measured facial indices for Vectra, Artec, and Sense with the respective P values when compared with Vectra

Abbreviation/Full Name	Vectra	Artec	P Value	Sense	P Value
Upper face-face height index	0.658 (0.02)	0.664 (0.01)	.367	0.675 (0.02	.328
Lower face-face height index	0.547 (0.03)	0.552 (0.03)	.180	0.542 (0.02	.542
Mandibula-face height index	0.361 (0.02)	0.373 (0.02)	.012	0.376 (0.02)	.004
Mandibula-upper face height index	0.562 (0.04)	0.584 (0.04)	.022	0.588 (0.04)	< .001
Mandibula-lower face height index	0.661 (0.04)	0.676 (0.02)	.021	0.693 (0.03)	< .001

significantly different with $P = .014$ and $P < .001$, respectively, when compared with the Vectra. The Sense measured the upper lip-upper face height index, the upper lip-mandible height index, vermilion-total lower lip height index, vermilion-cutaneous lower lip height index, cutaneous-total lower lip height index, and intercanthal-mouth width index statistically significantly different with $P = .011$, $P = .011$, $P = .026$, $P = .016$, $P = .002$, $P = .003$, and $P < .001$. respectively.

Intrascanner Comparison

Intrascanner comparison for all assessments showed a high correlation for the Vectra system (Inter-class correlation coefficient (ICC), 0.861; confidence interval [CI], 0.771–0.952) and Artec Eva (ICC, 0.889; CI, 0.783–0.910), but a moderate correlation for Sense (ICC, 0.486; CI, 0.230–0.660).

DISCUSSION

This study investigated predefined measurements in the face and indices, created by the predefined measurements in 3 different 3D scanner systems (Vectra, Artec, and Sense). The results revealed that even inexpensive 3D scanners such as the consumer device Sense 3D and the industrial Artec Eva scanner can be used for valid measurements in the facial area. The results of the analysis show that the 3D facial images taken by the Artec Eva camera are largely comparable with those of the Vectra system, whereas 3D images using the Sense yielded significant deviations, especially for more complex surfaces.

Comparing all direct landmark measurements derived from the reference system, a mean deviation of 0.13 ± 2.71 mm (range: −10.26 to 13.93 mm) was found for the Artec scanner and -0.19 ± 3.81 mm (range: −14.09 to 18.92 mm)

Table 5
Table showing the mean measured distances and indices (±1 standard deviation) for the nasal measurements for Vectra, Artec, and Sense with the respective P values when compared with Vectra

Abbreviation/Full Name	Vectra	Artec	P Value	Sense	P Value
Nasal index	0.540 (0.07)	0.558 (0.07)	.017	0.503 (0.07)	.002
Intercanthal-nasal width index	0.931 (0.11)	0.917 (0.09)	.315	1.042 (0.15) -	< .001
Nose-face height index	0.469 (0.02)	0.468 (0.03)	.811	0.477 (0.02)	.142
Nose-mouth width index	0.562 (0.04)	0.614 (0.06)	< .001	0.558 (0.06)	.783
Nose-upper face height index	0.729 (0.03)	0.733 (0.03)	.360	0.746 (0.03)	.013
Nasal bridge index	1.374 (0.06)	1.368 (0.06)	.471	1.343 (0.05)	.013
Interalar width	30.563 (2.88)	31.202 (3.42)	.038	28.507 (3.79)	< .001
Columella length	9.829 (2.17)	11.296 (2.46)	< .001	9.898 (2.53)	.842
Nasofrontal angle	141.798 (6.68)	141.479 (6.57)	.469	144.199 (5.87)	.008
Nasal tip protrusion width index	0.648 (0.07)	0.642 (0.09)	.710	0.691 (0.10)	.029
Nasal tip protrusion-nose height index	0.345 (0.02)	0.353 (0.03)	.173	0.343 (0.03)	.940

Table 6
Table showing the mean measured distances and indices (±1 standard deviation) for the perioral measurements for Vectra, Artec, and Sense with the respective P values when compared with Vectra

Abbreviation/Full Name	Vectra	Artec	P Value	Sense	P Value
Cutaneous-total upper lip height index	0.646 (0.07)	0.630 (0.08)	.393	0.664 (0.06)	0.189
Vermilion-total upper lip height index	0.380 (0.06)	0.412 (0.08)	.061	0.357 (0.04)	0.073
Vermilion height index	0.605 (0.15)	0.674 (0.19)	.083	0.546 (0.11)	0.077
Upper lip-upper face height index	0.289 (0.04)	0.279 (0.03)	.070	0.270 (0.03)	0.011
Lower lip-face height index	0.270 (0.03)	0.264 (0.03)	.236	0.277 (0.02)	0.252
Lower lip-mandible height index	0.398 (0.08)	0.394 (0.04)	.758	0.404 (0.04)	0.660
Upper lip height-mouth width index	0.417 (0.06)	0.423 (0.06)	.482	0.406 (0.07)	0.113
Vermilion-cutaneous upper lip height index	0.605 (0.15)	0.674 (0.19)	.084	0.546 (0.11)	0.077
Upper lip-mandible height index	0.516 (0.09)	0.478 (0.05)	.014	0.467 (0.08)	0.011
Lower-upper lip height index	0.805 (0.12)	0.824 (0.13)	.510	0.877 (0.11)	0.026
Cutaneous lower-upper lip height index	0.806 (0.16)	0.856 (0.13)	.115	0.778 (0.18)	0.335
Vermilion-total lower lip height index	0.426 (0.07)	0.432 (0.09)	.640	0.461 (0.09)	0.016
Vermilion-cutaneous lower lip height index	0.682 (0.17)	0.676 (0.21)	.855	0.829 (0.26)	0.002
Cutaneous-total lower lip height index	0.640 (0.06)	0.660 (0.07)	.131	0.583 (0.09)	0.003
Intercanthal-mouth width index	0.521 (0.05)	0.561 (0.06)	< .001	0.576 (0.06)	< 0.001

for the Sense scanner. In a similarly designed study, Weinberg and colleagues[21] compared 3D anthropometric measurements performed on mannequin heads, but without real-life test subjects. The results of Weinberg and colleagues[21] revealed that the differences in the linear distances consistently stayed less than 1 mm. Some differences in our study were greater than 1 mm for the Artec and the Sense 3D scanner; however, the examination of test subjects, when compared with lifeless mannequin heads, could increase the variability and error due to subtle changes in facial expression and more complex surface properties.[22] Moreover, de Menezes and colleagues[23] found that among repeated measurements of the facial area the results from the stationary Vectra system ranged from 0.13 to 1.19 mm.

In previous studies, an error of less than 2 mm was generally considered accurate and precise enough for the validation of 3D photogrammetry. However, a deviation of 1 to 2 mm may become relevant[12] in the clinical setting, for example,

when high-precision measurements are required; this is the case in maxillofacial surgery, in reconstructive and esthetic nose surgery, as well as in general facial surgery and especially in the assessment of postinterventional outcomes of soft tissue fillers.

Achieving harmony from cosmetic surgery often requires correcting disproportions. The proportions of the face and the absolute length of the facial structure are of immense value when it comes to assessing the facial profile of a patient in consultation, as well as in surgical planning and evaluation.[24] For this reason, we have included information on absolute face length and facial proportions. We could not show any statistical differences between the 3 scanners in the comparison of our 3D scanners. The variability was small. When compared with other studies, even the inexpensive scanner was able to display correct proportions.

The nose plays an integral role in the perception of facial attractiveness. Achieving angulations

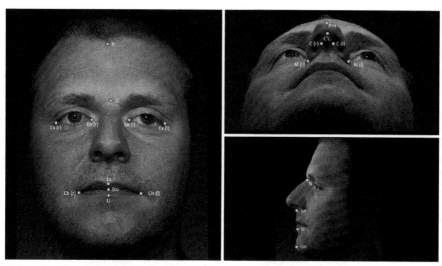

Fig. 1. Panel showing the respective landmarks used for the assessment of the respective distances and indices. Ex: Lateral canthus; En: Medial canthus; G: Glabella; Tr: Trichinion; Sto: Stoma; Ch: Cheilion; Ls: Superior lip; Li: Inferior Lip; Al: Ala; C: Columella; C'c: Columella center; N: Nasale; Sn: Subnasale; Gn: Gonium.

within norms for a given patient will help achieve an esthetically pleasing nose. Abnormalities in angulations and facial proportions appear much worse than minor asymmetries or shape irregularities. We were able to show that the measurements acquired with the 3 different 3D systems did not differ statistically significantly in most instances. The dimensions of the nose are also an important factor in the assessment of the nose.

The dimensions and proportions of the mouth and lips are an essential part of the symmetry and aesthetics of the face and a frequent target of noninvasive interventions such as soft tissue-based lip enhancement.[25] With all 3 scanners we were able to capture the classic proportions of the lip and dimensions of the mouth.

As practical guidance, it should be noted that for the best scanning results, the patient needs to

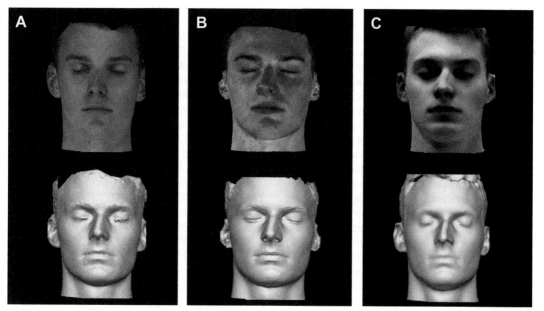

Fig. 2. Panel showing the frontal images acquired with the Vectra XT 3D Surface Imaging System (*A*), mobile Artec Eva scanner (*B*), and the mobile Sense 3D Scanner (*C*).

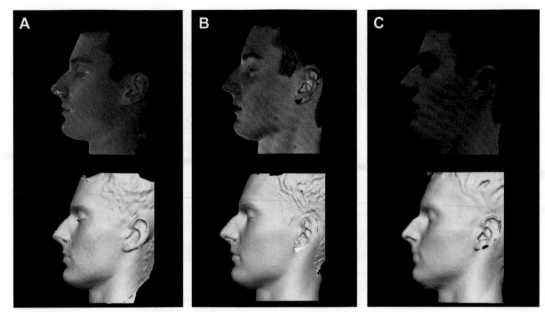

Fig. 3. Panel showing the lateral images acquired with the Vectra XT 3D Surface Imaging System (*A*), mobile Artec Eva scanner (*B*), and the mobile Sense 3D Scanner (*C*).

maintain a consistent position and facial expression throughout the recording process. Otherwise, motion artifacts could affect the final 3D model. The texture quality for Vectra and Artec Eva was excellent, whereas the textures of the Sense scanner were washed out and not representative of patient recordings; this can be seen in **Figs. 1–3**. Especially in esthetic consultations, this could have a negative impact on 3D patient counseling and, despite modest deviations, limits the usage of the 3D scanner for this application. An advantage for both portable devices is the mobile use of the camera in a variety of environments that is not limited to a particular stationary location. Potential locations for the use of the portable 3D scanners are the operating room, changing patient examination rooms in the clinic, and cross-location recordings.

Limitations of our study were the young volunteer collective investigated. Owing to limited age of the investigated volunteers, facial features such as severe rhytids or folds, which might be hard depict accurately by the 3D imaging systems, were not present in most volunteers. Moreover, the landmark measurement was automated using the Canfield Sculptor software. However, owing to the coarse surface and weak texture of the Sense Scanner, the landmark placement was occasionally incorrect and was corrected manually. In contrast to other studies, we did not investigate the variability in the study, because this has already been validated several times with the Canfield software. Despite automatic software-based landmark placement and verification by the examiner, examiner-dependent errors cannot be completely excluded.

Summary

This study investigated differences in facial acquisition and measurement between 3 different scans based on a relatively young and slim subject clientele. Especially for purely 2D distances as well as simple proportion and angle measurements, reliable measurements could be performed accurately by all investigated 3D systems. The results revealed that even with an affordable 3D scanner capturing the face and evaluating it using established classic measurements is, within mentioned limitations, possible.

CLINICS CARE POINTS

- Even inexpensive 3D scanners such as the consumer device Sense 3D and the industrial Artec Eva scanner can be used for valid measurements in the facial areaical guidance, it should be noted that for the best scanning results, the patient needs to maintain a consistent position and facial expression throughout the recording process.

AUTHOR DISCLOSURE

None of the other authors listed have any commercial associations or financial disclosures that might pose or create a conflict of interest with the methods applied or the results presented in this article.

REFERENCES

1. Koban K, Leitsch S, Holzbach T, et al. 3D bilderfassung und analyse in der plastischen chirurgie mit smartphone und tablet: eine alternative zu professionellen systemen? Handchir ·Mikrochir·Plast Chir. 2014;46(02):97–104.
2. Koban KC, Titze V, Etzel L, et al. Quantitative volumetric analysis of the lower extremity: Validation against established tape measurement and water displacement. Handchir Mikrochir Plast Chir 2018;50(6):393–9.
3. Freytag DL, Alfertshofer MG, Frank K, et al. The difference in facial movement between the medial and the lateral midface: a 3D skin surface vector analysis. Aesthet Surg J 2021. https://doi.org/10.1093/asj/sjab152.
4. Corey CL, Popelka GR, Barrera JE, et al. An analysis of malar fat volume in two age groups: implications for craniofacial surgery. Craniomaxillofac Trauma Reconstr 2012;5(4):231–4.
5. Koban KC, Härtnagl F, Titze V, et al. Chances and limitations of a low-cost mobile 3D scanner for breast imaging in comparison to an established 3D photogrammetric system. J Plast Reconstr Aesthet Surg 2018;71(10):1417–23.
6. Etzel L, Koban KC, Li Z, et al. [Whole-body surface assessment - implementation and experiences with 360° 3D whole-body scans: opportunities to objectively monitor the extremities and the body trunk]. Handchir Mikrochir Plast Chir 2019;51(4):240–8.
7. Cotofana S, Koban CK, Frank K, et al. The surface-volume-coefficient of the superficial and deep facial fat compartments – a cadaveric 3d volumetric analysis. Plast Reconstr Surg 2019;143(6):1605–13.
8. Koban KC, Titze V, Etzel L, et al. Quantitative volumetrische Analyse der unteren Extremität: Validierung gegenüber etablierter Maßbandmessung und Wasserverdrängung. Handchir ·Mikrochir ·Plast Chir. 2018;50(06):393–9.
9. Koban KC, Frank K, Etzel L, et al. 3D mammometric changes in the treatment of idiopathic gynecomastia. Aesthetic Plast Surg 2019;43(3):616–24.
10. Koban KC, Cotofana S, Frank K, et al. Precision in 3-Dimensional surface imaging of the face: a handheld scanner comparison performed in a cadaveric model. Aesthet Surg J 2019;39(4):NP36–44.
11. Koban KC, Leitsch S, Holzbach T, et al. [3D-imaging and analysis for plastic surgery by smartphone and tablet: an alternative to professional systems? Handchirurgie, Mikrochirurgie, Plast Chir 2014;46(2):97–104.
12. Koban KC, Perko P, Etzel L, et al. Validation of two handheld devices against a non-portable three-dimensional surface scanner and assessment of potential use for intraoperative facial imaging. J Plast Reconstr Aesthet Surg 2020;73(1):141–8.
13. Cotofana S, Koban K, Pavicic T, et al. Clinical validation of the surface volume coefficient for minimally invasive treatment of the temple. J Drugs Dermatol 2019;18(6):533. Available at: http://www.ncbi.nlm.nih.gov/pubmed/31251545.
14. Lekakis G, Claes P, Hamilton GS 3rd, et al. Three-dimensional surface imaging and the continuous evolution of preoperative and postoperative assessment in rhinoplasty. Facial Plast Surg 2016;32(1):88–94.
15. Koban K, Schenck T, Giunta R. Using Mobile 3D Scanning Systems for Objective Evaluation of Form, Volume, and Symmetry in Plastic Surgery: Intraoperative Scanning and Lymphedema Assessment. Deutsche Gesellschaft für Plastische und Rekonstruktive Chirurgie Jahreskongress 2016.
16. Haidar R, Freytag DL, Frank K, et al. Quantitative analysis of the lifting effect of facial soft-tissue filler injections. Plast Reconstr Surg 2021;147:765e–76e.
17. Alfertshofer M, Frank K, Melnikov DV, et al. Performing Distance measurements in curved facial regions: a comparison between three-dimensional surface scanning and ultrasound imaging. Facial Plast Surg 2021. https://doi.org/10.1055/s-0041-1725166.
18. Hernandez CA, Freytag DL, Gold MH, et al. Clinical validation of the temporal lifting technique using soft tissue fillers. J Cosmet Dermatol 2020. https://doi.org/10.1111/jocd.13621. jocd.13621.
19. Frank K, Freytag DL, Schenck TL, et al. Relationship between forehead motion and the shape of forehead lines-A 3D skin displacement vector analysis. J Cosmet Dermatol 2019. https://doi.org/10.1111/jocd.13065.
20. WMA Declaration of Helsinki – Ethical Principles for Medical Research Involving Human Subjects – WMA – The World Medical Association. Available at: https://www.wma.net/policies-post/wma-declaration-of-helsinki-ethical-principles-for-medical-research-involving-human-subjects/. Accessed August 5, 2018.
21. Weinberg SM, Naidoo S, Govier DP, et al. Anthropometric precision and accuracy of digital three-dimensional photogrammetry: comparing the Genex and 3dMD imaging systems with one another and with direct anthropometry. J Craniofac Surg 2006;17(3):477–83.

22. TJJ Maal, Verhamme LM, van Loon B, et al. Variation of the face in rest using 3D stereophotogrammetry. Int J Oral Maxillofac Surg 2011;40(11):1252–7.

23. de Menezes M, Rosati R, Ferrario VF, et al. Accuracy and Reproducibility of a 3-Dimensional Stereophotogrammetric Imaging System. J Oral Maxillofac Surg 2010;68(9):2129–35.

24. Milutinovic J, Zelic K, Nedeljkovic N. Evaluation of facial beauty using anthropometric proportions. ScientificWorldJournal 2014;2014:428250.

25. Kar M, Muluk NB, Bafaqeeh SA, et al. Is it possible to define the ideal lips? Acta Otorhinolaryngol Ital 2018. https://doi.org/10.14639/0392-100X-1511.

26. Farkas LG, Tompson B, Phillips JH, et al. Comparison of anthropometric and cephalometric measurements of the adult face. J Craniofac Surg 1999; 10(1):18–25 [discussion: 26].

27. Swennen GRJ, Schutyser F, Hausamen JE, et al. Three-dimensional cephalometry: a color atlas and manual 2006. https://doi.org/10.1007/3-540-29011-7.

Accuracy Assessment of Three-Dimensional Surface Imaging–Based Distance Measurements of the Face

Comparison of a Handheld Facial Scanner and a Stationary Whole-Body Surface Imaging Device

Konstantin Christoph Koban, MD[a], Ya Xu, MD[a], Nicholas Moellhoff, MD[a], Denis Ehrl, MD, PhD[a], Michael G. Alfertshofer[a], Sebastian Cotofana, MD, PhD[b], Riccardo E. Giunta, MD, PhD[a], Julie Woodward, MD, PhD[c], Daria Voropai, MD[d], Konstantin Frank, MD[a],*

KEYWORDS

• 3D scan • Face scan • Whole-body scan • Surface imaging • Whole-body imaging

INTRODUCTION

Three-dimensional surface imaging (3DSI) has been shown to be a useful tool for plastic surgeons in the preoperative, intraoperative, and postoperative setting.[1–12] Volumetric and spatial changes after body-contouring surgeries such as breast augmentation, abdominoplasties, liposuctions, and lipofilling or minimally invasive treatments such as soft tissue filler augmentations can be objectively recorded using 3DSI.[9,13–18] A myriad of 3DSI devices has evolved since their introduction in 1967 by Burke and Beard and developed into 2 directions.[6] On the one hand, 3-dimensional surface imaging devices have become more versatile, handy, lighter, and easy to use (ie, handheld devices); on the other hand 3DSI devices evolved to capture the entire body, rather than only one, are of interest (ie, whole-body scanner).[5,19]

Handheld devices are light, easy to use, and often at a lower price than whole-body imaging devices. Potential drawbacks of imaging devices that capture the entire body are a high price and a large uptake of space in the case of permanently installed systems. The question remains whether whole-body surface acquisition with high texture quality comes at the cost of a loss of quality in more geometric complex areas such as the facial region, which is required for accurate volumetric and spatial measurements. Especially surgical and minimally invasive interventions in the face cause small volumetric and spatial changes, which however have a great effect on the patient's appearance. Thus, accurate and high-resolution 3DSI are inevitable for a proper follow-up and also for scientific purposes.[1,5] As clinicians and researchers rely on accurate measurements, the accuracy of handheld devices should be compared

Funding: This study received no funding
[a] Department for Hand, Plastic and Aesthetic Surgery, Ludwig – Maximilian University Munich, Munich, Germany; [b] Department of Clinical Anatomy, Mayo Clinic College of Medicine and Science, Rochester, MN, USA; [c] Duke University Medical Center, Durham, NC, USA; [d] Private Practice, Amsterdam, the Netherlands
* Corresponding author. Division for Hand, Plastic and Aesthetic Surgery, Ludwig – Maximilian University Munich, Pettenkoferstraße 8A, Munich 80336, Germany
E-mail address: konstantin.frank@med.uni-muenchen.de

Facial Plast Surg Clin N Am 30 (2022) 159–166
https://doi.org/10.1016/j.fsc.2022.01.009
1064-7406/22/© 2022 Elsevier Inc. All rights reserved.

with whole-body scanners to objectively advise which imaging device should be used in which instance. To the knowledge of the authors no 3-dimensional whole-body surface imaging system has been compared with a 3-dimensional hand-held surface imaging system so far. Thus, the objective of this investigation was to compare the accuracy of distance measurements in the face using a handheld surface imaging device and a whole-body surface imaging device.

MATERIALS AND METHODS
Study Sample

This investigation enrolled a total of 22 healthy volunteer (12 Caucasian, 10 Asian) with a mean age of 29.36 ± 7.7 years and a mean body mass index of 22.31 ± 1.5 kg/m^2. Participants were not enrolled in this study if previous facial surgeries, trauma, or diseases disrupted the integrity of the facial anatomy or major surface irregularities, as tattoos or permanent makeup were present. Volunteers were taught on the methods and scopes of this investigation before enrollment. Volunteers were asked to sign a provided written informed consent for the use of their data and captured images before enrollment into the investigation. This investigation was reviewed and approved by the Institutional Review Board of Ludwig-Maximilian University Munich (IRB protocol number: 266-13). The study was performed in accordance with regional laws (Germany) and good clinical practice.

IMAGING

Before imaging, a standard reference in the form of a 6 mm × 38 mm Steri-Strip (3M Deutschland GmbH, Neuss, Germany) was placed in the forehead, on the midface (bilateral), and on the lower face (midline). Steri-Strip size was controlled using a caliper before attachment. Afterward, 3-dimensional surface images of the faces of the participants using a Vectra H2 hand held camera system (Canfield Scientific Inc., Fairfield, New Jersey, USA) and whole-body images using the WB360 system (Canfield Scientific Inc., Fairfield, New Jersey, USA) were captured. The Vectra H2 and WB360 scanner use passive stereophotogrammetry to reconstruct 3-dimensional models obtained from digital photographs. Volunteers were asked to stand upright with a resting, relaxed face. Participants were asked to maintain their facial expression over the duration of the image acquisition. Volunteers removed jewelry to allow for optimal imaging of the face. After acquisition of the photographs, scans were processed using the Vectra Software Suite (Canfield Scientific Inc., Fairfield, New Jersey, USA).

IMAGE ANALYSES

The following distance measurements were performed in each scan (**Figs. 1** and **2**):

1) Length and width of the photographed steri-strip on the forehead
2) Length and width of the photographed steri-strip on the midface (bilateral)
3) Length and width of the photographed steri-strip on the lower face

STATISTICAL ANALYSES

The difference to the length of the standard reference was calculated for each of the images obtained with the 2 investigated surface imaging devices (H2 vs WB360) and compared via a paired Student's t-test. Differences between the length and width of the standard reference and the measured length and width were calculated as relative and absolute values and compared using Student's t-test. Analyses were performed using SPSS Statistics 23 (IBM, Armonk, NY, USA), and differences were considered statistically significant at a probability level of less than or equal to 0.05 to guide conclusions.

RESULTS

The average difference between the length and width of the standard reference and the measured

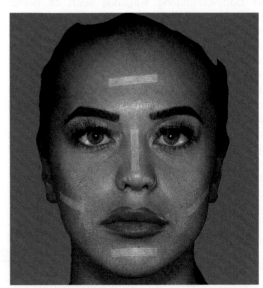

Fig. 1. The 3DSI photograph of a 25-year-old female participant with the attached steri-strips at the forehead, the midface, and the lower face acquired with the handheld 3DSI device.

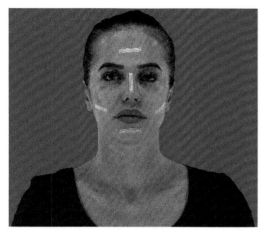

Fig. 2. The 3DSI photograph of a 25-year-old female participant with the attached steri-strips at the forehead, the midface, and the lower face acquired with the stationary whole-body imaging device.

different investigated areas of the face was found for measured lengths and widths ($P < .001$).

FOREHEAD MEASUREMENTS

The average difference between length of the standard reference and the measured length in the forehead was -0.29 ± 0.3 mm for the H2 and $-0.40 + 0.5$ mm for the WB360 ($P = .422$). The average difference between width of the standard reference and the measured width was 0.32 ± 0.2 mm for the H2 and $0.43 + 0.2$ mm for the WB360 ($P = .032$). Paired samples t-test revealed a significant difference between the length of the standard reference and the measured length for both the H2 and the WB360 with $P = .001$ and $P = .002$, respectively, and between the width of the standard reference and the measured width $P < .001$ for both H2 and WB360 (**Figs. 3** and **4**) (**Tables 1-4**)

length and width, independent of investigated facial area (forehead vs midface vs lower face) or investigated surface imaging device, was -0.56 ± 0.9 mm and 0.33 ± 0.2 mm, respectively. Independent of facial region, the mean difference to the standard reference of the measured length was -0.65 ± 0.8 mm for the H2 imaging device and -0.46 ± 1.0 mm for the WB360 imaging device with $P = .112$. Independent of facial region, the mean difference to the standard reference of the measured width was 0.29 ± 0.1 mm for the H2 imaging device and 0.37 ± 0.3 mm for the WB360 imaging device with $P = .017$. A significant difference between the differences across the

MIDFACE MEASUREMENTS

The average difference between length of the standard reference and the measured length in the midface was -0.35 ± 0.4 mm for the H2 and $-0.21 + 0.7$ mm for the WB360 ($P = .266$). The average difference between width of the standard reference and the measured width was 0.28 ± 0.2 mm for the H2 and $0.50 + 0.2$ mm for the WB360 ($P < .001$). Paired samples t-test revealed a significant difference between the length of the standard reference and the measured length for both the H2 and the WB360 with $P < .001$ and $P = .048$, respectively, and between

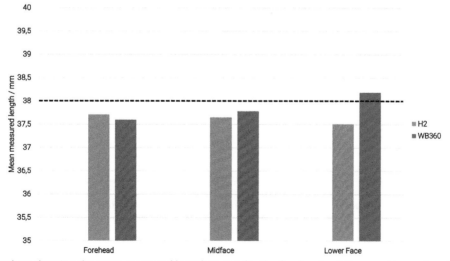

Fig. 3. Bar chart showing the mean measured length in mm for the forehead, midface, and lower face for the H2 and WB360, respectively.

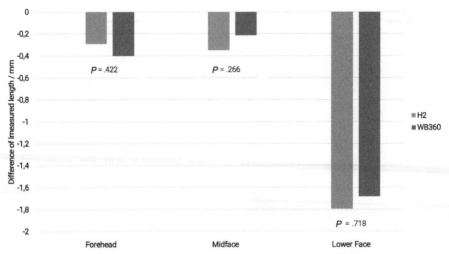

Fig. 4. Bar chart showing the average difference between the length of the standard reference and the measured length for the H2 and WB360. P-values between the 2 camera systems are given.

Table 1
The mean difference between length of the standard reference and the measured length in mm for the respective location and the respective imaging device

Forehead		Midface		Lower Face	
H2	WB360	H2	WB360	H2	WB360
0.29 ± 0.4	0.40 ± 0.5	$0.35 + 0.4$	$0.21 + 0.7$	1.80 ± 1.0	1.68 ± 1.1
$P = .422$		$P = .266$		$P = .718$	

P-values for the difference between the respective imaging devices are given.

Table 2
The mean difference between width of the standard reference and the measured length in mm for the respective location and the respective imaging device

Forehead		Midface		Lower Face	
H2	WB360	H2	WB360	H2	WB360
-0.32 ± 0.2	-0.43 ± 0.2	-0.28 ± 0.2	-0.50 ± 0.2	-0.28 ± 0.1	-0.43 ± 0.1
$P = .032$		$P < .001$		$P < .001$	

P-values for the difference between the respective imaging devices are given

Table 3
P-values for differences between the length of the standard reference and the measured length

Forehead		Midface		Lower Face	
H2	WB360	H2	WB360	H2	WB360
$P = .001$	$P = .002$	$P < .001$	$P = .048$	$P < .001$	$P < .001$

Table 4
P-values for differences between the width of the standard reference and the measured length

Forehead		Midface		Lower Face	
H2	WB360	H2	WB360	H2	WB360
$P < .001$	$P < .001$	$P < .001$	$P < .001$	$P < .001$	$P < .001$

the width of the standard reference and the measured width $P < .001$ for both H2 and WB360 (**Fig. 5**).

LOWER FACE MEASUREMENTS

The average difference between length of the standard reference and the measured length in the lower face was -1.80 ± 1.0 mm for the H2 and $-1.68 + 1.1$ mm for the WB360 ($P = .718$). The average difference between width of the standard reference and the measured width was 0.28 ± 0.1 mm for the H2 and $0.43 + 0.1$ mm for the WB360 ($P < .001$). Paired samples t-test revealed a significant difference between the length of the standard reference and the measured length for both the H2 and the WB360 with $P < .001$ and between the width of the standard reference and the measured width $P < .001$ for the H2 and WB360 (**Fig. 6**).

DISCUSSION

This study investigated the accuracy of facial 3DSI scans obtained with a handheld imaging device (Vectra H2) and a whole-body imaging device (WB360) by comparing the measurements obtained from the scans to a standard reference, which was a 38×6 mm-sized steri-strip attached to various regions in the face of 22 individuals. Our results revealed that the measured difference between the length and the standard reference did not differ statistically significant between the 2 investigated devices in all investigated areas of the face ($P > .266$); however, the measured difference of the width and the width of the standard reference differed statistically significant in all areas of the face ($P < .032$). When testing for statistical significance, the obtained measurements (both length and width) from the 3DSI scans differed significantly from the standard reference in all areas of the face for both imaging devices (H2 and WB360) with $P < .048$.

A strength of this study is the constant testing environment. Images of the subjects were photographed under the same lighting conditions. As images were captured with both imaging systems immediately after each other, altered mimic, local swelling or movement artifacts could be excluded. Because all data were obtained by the same investigator (Y.X.), consistency could be provided and observer-dependent bias was negated. Furthermore, using standard references allowed to objectively assess whether the obtained measurements from the 3DSI over- or underestimated the respective lengths and widths. Furthermore, a sample

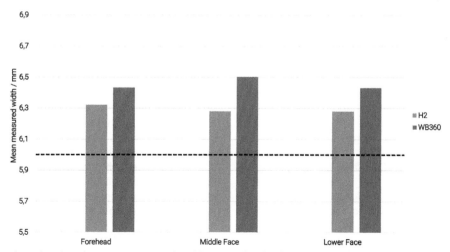

Fig. 5. Bar chart showing the mean measured width in mm for the forehead, midface, and lower face for the H2 and WB360, respectively.

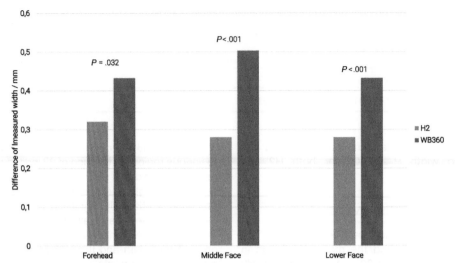

Fig. 6. Bar chart showing the average difference between the width of the standard reference and the measured length for the H2 and WB360. P-values between the 2 camera systems are given.

size of 22 participants with 4 applied standard references yielded a total of 98 observations, which is to the knowledge of the authors the biggest sample size that was investigated to validate and compare measurements of a handheld and whole-body 3DSI device. Although many 3DSI systems require a calibration before image capture, which needs to be performed by the user, the investigated camera systems perform a self-calibration with updated internal calibrations files, which further reduces technical error during the capturing of the image. However, the authors want to point out that naturally a complete eradication of technical errors can never be ruled out.

A potential drawback of this study is the standard reference itself. Even though steri-strips were not manipulated and checked with a caliper, this study relied on the manufacturer's details about length and width of the produced steri-strips. The caliper measurements used did not show any difference between the stated size; however, even if proper attachment was performed in all instances, minimal crimping or elongation of the steri-strip, which might affect the measurement results, could not be completely ruled out. Furthermore, adhesion of the steri-strips might differ in-between the image capturing with the H2 and the WB360 due to transpiration of the individual. Another potential drawback of this investigation is the lack of capturing volumetric changes. Especially in the follow-up of treatments with soft tissue fillers or autologous lipofilling volumetric changes are important. Our study did not include any volumetric changes, which might limit the clinical application of its findings; however, the authors have the strong view that spatial distance

measurements are of inevitable importance in the clinical and research field.

Interestingly, the measurements of the length of the standard reference were most accurate in the midface when captured with the WB360 and least accurate in the lower face when captured with the H2. A possible explanation for this might be the diminished cohesivity of the steri-strips on the hairy lower face of men, which might have consecutively caused the steri-strip to be offstanding and minimally overlapping. Physicians should thus keep in mind that facial hair might disrupt the integrity and accuracy of a 3DSI scan and furthermore limit its evaluability. This finding is in line with recent findings by Koban and colleagues that found the greatest variation within scans to be at the mouth and the eye region.[19]

Another finding of this investigation is that the measured length of the steri-strips was in general greater, whereas the measured width of the steri-strips was in average smaller. Practitioners should thus keep in mind that vertical measurements might be underestimated when using both 3DSI devices, whereas horizontal measurements might likely be overstated. At the same time, it needs to be pointed out that 3DSI has shown to be of less precision when it comes to assessing small distances. Especially in the follow-up of small spatial distances, that is, after rhinoplasties or even in the setting of studies investigating minimally invasive procedures, this potential limitation should be pointed out and communicated to the user.

The measured difference between length of the standard reference and the measured length was greater for the H2 than for the WB360 except at the forehead; this can be attributed to the creation of the image. The WB360 captures the body with 92 fixed installed cameras, and the only source of error, that is, changes in the face of the scanned individual, are caused by movement of the individual itself. Capturing a 3DSI with the H2 requires the investigator to take a face capture at a 45° angle from the front toward the right side of the face at the patient's chest level, directly in front of the face at the level of the patient's face not angled, and at a 45° angle from the front toward the left side of the face at the patient's chest level. Simultaneously, 2 red dots need to be converged to allow for the optimal focus of the images taken. Even when painstakingly aiming to reproduce the same distances and angles, this process is a source for human error in the capturing process. Additional to the aforementioned human error in the capturing process on the investigator's side, the same movement artifacts caused by the captured participant add to possible deviations. Practitioners should be aware that using handheld 3DSI devices adds a further source or error to the capturing process, compared with stationary 3DSI devices.

Even though p-values for differences between the length and width of the standard reference and the measured length and width were statistically highly significant in all investigated areas, it needs to be pointed out that the absolute difference ranged from −1.14 to 4.3 mm. Although statistically significant different, the divergence from the standard reference should still be considered acceptable. Clinical follow-up and follow-up imaging sessions in the research field require accurate acquisition; however, the, although statistically significant, deviations should be considered as acceptable. The question whether 3DSI is overall superior to measuring spatial distances in classic 2-dimensional photographs is worthy to be discussed. Although spatial distances can be assessed using 2-dimensional photographs, a referencing needs to be placed onto the skin of the face of the captured person; this is on one hand uncomfortable and impractical, whereas on the other hand does not take depth and curvature into account. Thus, the lack of depth into the capturing measurements taken using classic 2-dimensional photography will be with a very high probability less accurate than using 3DSI.

SUMMARY

Measurements obtained from scans acquired using the handheld imaging device and the whole-body imaging device both differed significantly from the standard reference. However, the absolute differences were small. We thus conclude that physicians and researchers should be aware of deviations when obtaining 3DSI using the presented imaging devices but should not refrain from using them, as the absolute differences might be too small to play a role in both, clinical and research, settings.

CLINICS CARE POINTS

- Measurements from scans using a handheld imaging device and a whole-body imaging device both differed significantly from the standard reference.
- Physicians and researchers should be aware of deviations when obtaining 3DSI using the presented imaging devices.
- Absolute differences might be too small to play a role in both, clinical and research, settings.

AUTHOR DISCLOSURE

None of the other authors listed have any commercial associations or financial disclosures that might pose or create a conflict of interest with the methods applied or the results presented in this article.

REFERENCES

1. Cotofana S, Koban K, Pavicic T, et al. Clinical Validation of the surface volume coefficient for minimally invasive treatment of the temple. J Drugs Dermatol 2019;18(6):533. Available at: http://www.ncbi.nlm.nih.gov/pubmed/31251545. Accessed August 13, 2019.
2. Cotofana S, Gotkin RH, Frank K, et al. Anatomy behind the facial overfilled syndrome: the transverse facial septum. Dermatol Surg 2019. https://doi.org/10.1097/DSS.0000000000002236.
3. Casabona G, Frank K, Koban KC, et al. Lifting vs volumizing-the difference in facial minimally invasive procedures when respecting the line of ligaments. J Cosmet Dermatol 2019. https://doi.org/10.1111/jocd.13089.
4. Koban K, Schenck T, Metz P, et al. Auf dem Weg zur objektiven Evaluation von Form, Volumen und Symmetrie in der Plastischen Chirurgie mittels intraoperativer 3D Scans. Handchirurgie · Mikrochirurgie · Plast Chir 2016;48(02):78–84.
5. Koban KC, Cotofana S, Frank K, et al. Precision in 3-dimensional surface imaging of the face: a handheld

scanner comparison performed in a cadaveric model. Aesthet Surg J 2019;39(4):NP36–44.

6. Cotofana S, Koban CK, Frank K, et al. The Surface-volume-coefficient of the superficial and deep facial fat compartments – a cadaveric 3d volumetric analysis. Plast Reconstr Surg 2019;143(6):1.

7. Frank K, Freytag DL, Schenck TL, et al. Relationship between forehead motion and the shape of forehead lines—a 3D skin displacement vector analysis. J Cosmet Dermatol 2019;18(5):1224–9.

8. Cotofana S, Freytag DL, Frank K, et al. The Bi-directional movement of the frontalis muscle - introducing the line of convergence and its potential clinical relevance. Plast Reconstr Surg 2020. https://doi.org/10.1097/PRS.0000000000006756.

9. Koban KC, Frank K, Etzel L, et al. 3D mammometric changes in the treatment of idiopathic gynecomastia. Aesthet Plast Surg 2019;43(3):616–24.

10. Etzel L, Koban KC, Li Z, et al. [Whole-body surface assessment - implementation and experiences with 360° 3D whole-body scans: opportunities to objectively monitor the extremities and the body trunk]. Handchir Mikrochir Plast Chir 2019;51(4):240–8.

11. Koban KC, Titze V, Etzel L, et al. Quantitative volumetric analysis of the lower extremity: validation against established tape measurement and water displacement. Handchirurgie Mikrochirurgie Plast Chir 2018;50(6):393–9.

12. Koban KC, Härtnagl F, Titze V, et al. Chances and limitations of a low-cost mobile 3D scanner for breast imaging in comparison to an established 3D photogrammetric system. J Plast Reconstr Aesthet Surg 2018. https://doi.org/10.1016/j.bjps.2018.05.017.

13. Rieger UM, Erba P, Wettstein R, et al. Does abdominoplasty with liposuction of the love handles yield a shorter scar? An analysis with abdominal 3D laser scanning. Ann Plast Surg 2008 Oct;61(4):359–63. https://doi.org/10.1097/SAP.0b013e31816d824a.

14. Spanholtz T, Leitsch S, Holzbach T, et al. 3-dimensionale Bilderfassung: Erste Erfahrungen in der Planung und Dokumentation plastisch-chirurgischer Operationen. Handchirurgie Mikrochirurgie · Plast Chir 2012;44(04):234–9.

15. Frank K, Koban K, Targosinski S, et al. The anatomy behind adverse events in hand volumizing procedures. Plast Reconstr Surg 2018;141(5):650e–62e.

16. Chae MP, Rozen WM, Spychal RT, et al. Breast volumetric analysis for aesthetic planning in breast reconstruction: a literature review of techniques. Gland Surg 2016;5(2):212–26.

17. de Runz A, Boccara D, Bertheuil N, et al. Three-dimensional imaging, an important factor of decision in breast augmentation. Ann Chir Plast Esthet 2017. https://doi.org/10.1016/j.anplas.2017.07.019.

18. Koban KC, Etzel L, Li Z, et al. Three-dimensional surface imaging in breast cancer: A new tool for clinical studies? Radiat Oncol 2020;15(1). https://doi.org/10.1186/s13014-020-01499-2.

19. Koban KC, Perko P, Etzel L, et al. Validation of two handheld devices against a non-portable three-dimensional surface scanner and assessment of potential use for intraoperative facial imaging. J Plast Reconstr Aesthet Surg 2020;73(1):141–8.

Anatomic Differences Between the Asian and Caucasian Nose and Their Implications for Liquid Rhinoplasties

Zhouxiao Li, MD[a], Konstantin Frank, MD[a], Lukas H. Kohler, MD[a],
Nicholas Moellhoff, MD[a], Riccardo E. Giunta, MD[a],
Sebastian Cotofana, MD, PhD[b], Michael G. Alfertshofer[a],
Julie Woodward, MD[c], Daria Voropai, MD[d],
Konstantin Christoph Koban, MD[a],*

KEYWORDS

- Liquid rhinoplasties • Ethnic differences • Caucasians • Asians • Soft tissue fillers

INTRODUCTION

The demand for nose augmentations using minimally invasive interventions, majorly by injecting hyaluronic acid–based soft-tissue fillers, has spiked in the last decades. The American Society of Aesthetic Plastic Surgeons reported an increase of 26.4% since 2015 for soft-tissue augmentations in the face, whereas a decrease of 3.7% since 2015 was reported for surgical rhinoplasties.[1] Quick procedure times, short downtimes after the intervention, comparably less swelling and bruising, reversibility using hyaluronidase, as well as less pain are advantages of minimally invasive interventions using hyaluronic acid–based soft-tissue fillers when compared with classical rhinoplasties.[2–4] Despite numerous advantages, potential drawbacks, limitations, and adverse events need to be discussed with the patient seeking correction of the nose. Although surgical rhinoplasties allow to sculpt the nose in a holistic way

because of the possibility to add and reduce volume, approaching nasal deformities with soft-tissue fillers, also known as liquid rhinoplasties, is rather limited, as only volume can be added, but not removed. This limits the versatility of liquid rhinoplasties, while at the same time challenges the practitioner to precisely know the nasal anatomy and topography of the nose to perform corrections without removing excessive bone, cartilage, or fat.

Recent investigations have shown that significant changes exist between the underlying anatomy of the nose in Caucasians and Asians.[5,6] This consecutively affects the topographic 3-dimensional appearance of the nose. As practitioners are commonly frequented by patients from a wide array of ethnicities, injection protocols and schemes need to be adjusted to create satisfactory results. Thus, the objective of this investigation was to assess morphologic differences between Asians and Caucasians using 3-dimensional surface imaging. It is hoped that the results

Funding: No funding needs to be reported for this investigation.
[a] Department for Hand, Plastic and Aesthetic Surgery, Ludwig – Maximilian University Munich, Germany;
[b] Department of Clinical Anatomy, Mayo Clinic College of Medicine and Science, Rochester, MN, USA;
[c] Duke University Medical Center, Durham, NC, USA; [d] Private Practice, Amsterdam, Netherlands
* Corresponding author. Division for Hand, Plastic and Aesthetic Surgery Ludwig – Maximilian University Munich, Germany, Pettenkoferstraße 8A, Munich 80336, Germany.
E-mail address: konstantin.koban@med.uni-muenchen.de

Facial Plast Surg Clin N Am 30 (2022) 167–173
https://doi.org/10.1016/j.fsc.2022.01.008

can be used as guidance for practitioners when performing liquid rhinoplasties on patients from different ethnicities.

MATERIAL AND METHODS
Study Sample

The investigated study sample consisted of 160 healthy participants (80 men, 80 women) with a mean age of 30.41 ± 4.5 years. Of those, 40 men and 40 women were of Asian ethnicity and 40 men and 40 women were of Caucasian ethnicity. Participants were recruited at the outpatient department of the REDACTED. Before initiation of the study, participants were screened and not included in this investigation if a history of previous minimally invasive injections of soft-tissue fillers or neuromodulator treatments had been reported. Other criteria for exclusion were epilepsy, prior facial surgeries, facial trauma, or any type of disease or condition that could possibly affect the integrity of the facial anatomy. Participants were informed about the aims and procedures of the study (3-dimensional imaging). Each participant provided written informed consent for the use of both their data and associated images before enrollment. The study was approved by the Institutional Review Board of REDACTED (IRB protocol number: REDACTED). This investigation was conducted in accordance with regional laws maintaining good clinical practice.

3-Dimensional surface imaging

Facial 3-dimensional imaging was performed using a Vectra H2 camera (Canfield Scientific Inc, Fairfield, NJ, USA) to evaluate the nasal morphology of the participants. Participants were asked to remove any jewelry, glasses, and hair before 3-dimensional imaging. Imaging was performed in the same room with participants positioned in the same posture under identical lighting settings. Obtained surface scans were imported and processed in the Mirror Software Suite (Canfield Scientific Inc, Fairfield, NJ, USA). All measurements were conducted by the same investigator (Z.L.). The following morphometric parameters were evaluated and reported in mm for distances and degrees for angles:

- Face length and width
- Nasal length
- Nasal root width
- Dorsal bridge width at narrowest point
- Nasal base width
- Nasofrontal angle
- Nasal dorsum angle
- Nasolabial angle
- Glabella-nasion-sellion surface length

- Dorsum surface length
- Dorsum length

Descriptions of the measurements performed are given in **Figs. 1–3** and **Table 1**.

Statistical Analyses

Differences between measurements (Asian vs Caucasian; men vs women) were calculated using independent Student t test. Analyses were performed using SPSS Statistics 27 (IBM, Armonk, NY, USA) and differences were considered statistically significant at a probability level of ≤.05 to guide conclusions.

RESULTS
General Findings

Statistically significant differences between men and women, independent of ethnicity, were found for the face length and width, nasal length, narrowest dorsal bridge width, nasal base width, dorsum surface length, and dorsum length with $P < .003$. No statistically significant correlations between age and the measured parameters were found. Mean values for the entire study population are given in **Table 2**. Mean face length in Asians was 193.02 ± 9.6 mm and 186.19 ± 10.0 mm in Caucasians with $P < .001$, whereas mean face width was 177.10 ± 12.5 mm in Asians and 170.52 ± 14.1 mm in Caucasians with $P = .002$.

Nasal Width and Length—Ethnic Differences

The mean nasal length was 72.36 ± 4.8 mm in Asians and 66.59 ± 4.2 mm in Caucasians with $P < .001$. When adjusting to overall face length by creating a nose length–to–face length index, this difference remained statistically significantly different with $P < .001$ and a nose length–to–face length index of 0.38 ± 0.0 and 0.36 ± 0.0 for Asians and Caucasians, respectively. The nasal root width did not differ statistically significant between Asians and Caucasians with $P = .847$ and 25.91 ± 3.3 mm and 26.03 ± 4.4, respectively. The narrowest dorsal bridge width was 11.31 ± 1.8 mm in Asians and 14.67 ± 2.4 mm in Caucasians with $P < .001$. The dorsum surface length averaged at 43.95 ± 4.2 mm in Asians and 45.78 ± 4.0 mm in Caucasians with $P = .006$. The glabella-nasion-sellion length had an average length of 22.02 ± 3.0 mm in Asians and 15.35 ± 2.3 mm in Caucasians with $P < .001$. The nasal base had a mean width of 36.63 ± 2.8 mm in Asians and 30.61 ± 3.0 mm in Caucasians with $P < .001$. Gender differences are given in **Table 3**.

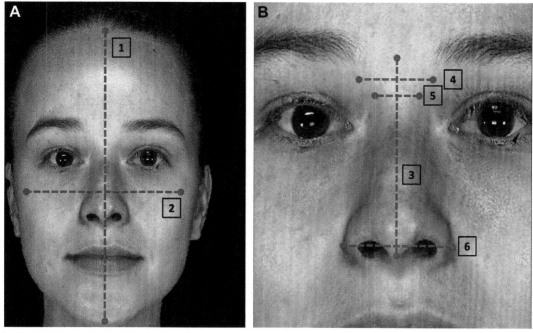

Fig. 1. *(A, B)* Frontal view (0°) of a female study participant depicting the measurement of facial length and width (1 and 2) in the left side and the measurement of nasal length (3), nasal root width (4), dorsal bridge width (5), and nasal base width (6) in the right side of the figure.

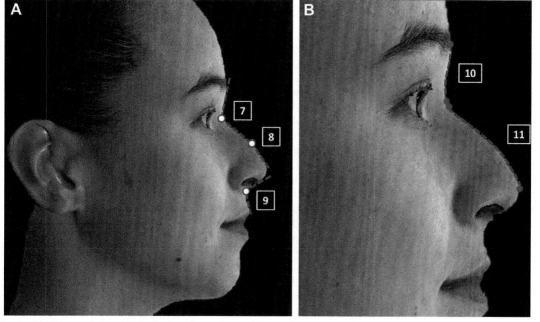

Fig. 2. *(A, B)* Lateral view (90°) of a female study participant depicting the measurement of the nasofrontal angle (7), the nasal dorsum angle (8), and the nasolabial angle (9) in the left side of the image and the Glabella-nasion-sellion surface length (10) as well as the dorsum surface length (11) in the right side of the figure.

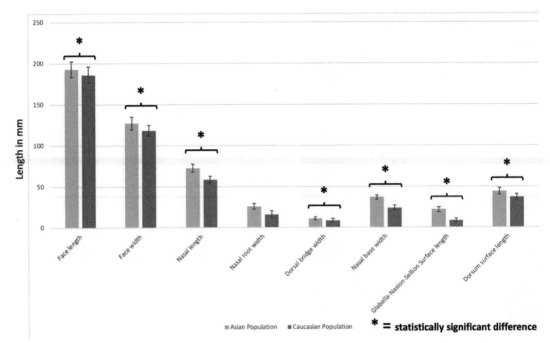

Fig. 3. Bar graph showing the mean values and standard deviation of the measured lengths and widths. Asterisks (*) indicate a statistically significant difference between the Asian and Caucasian population.

Nasal Angles

The nasolabial angle was on average 116.06° ± 10.7° in Asians and 117.97° ± 98° in Caucasians with $P < .001$. The nasofrontal angle was on average 145.84° ± 5.2° in Asians and 143.86° ± 6.3° with $P = .033$, whereas the nasal dorsum angle was 173.65° ± 5.2° in Asians and 174.80° ± 2.9° in Caucasians with $P = .088$.

DISCUSSION

This investigation compared the surface morphology of the nose in 80 Caucasians and 80 Asians using 3-dimensional surface imaging with reproducible clinical landmarks. The results revealed an overall high number of statistically different measurements. Interestingly, the nose of Asians was statistically significantly longer than the nose of Caucasians, even when adjusted for facial height, the narrowest dorsal bridge width was statistically smaller in Asians than in Caucasians and the nasal base statistically larger, whereas the dorsal surface length was longer in Caucasians than in Asians.

A common goal of liquid rhinoplasties is a tip correction of the nose, which is created by injecting soft-tissue filler into the columella base and altering the nasolabial angle. The ideal nasolabial angle was defined by Armijo and colleagues to be between 93.4° and 98.5° for men and 95.5° to

100.1° for women.[7] By supporting the columella base and adding volume to this region, the nasolabial angle is changed. An optic elevation of the tip is created if volume is added close to the subnasale, whereas an optic lowering of the tip is achieved by injecting more toward the tip itself along the columella. When investigating the nasolabial angle between Asians and Caucasians within men and women, our results are partially in line with previous reports. Gu and colleagues reported that the nasolabial angle, measured in lateral cephalograms, is smaller in Asian males and females when compared with Caucasian males and females. Although the absolute difference between Caucasian and Asian males was greater in our study sample, the absolute reported difference was approximately equal between Asian and Caucasian females.[8] Injectors should thus rely on individual assessment of the nasolabial angle and the position of the nasal tip and keep in mind that based on our findings, Asian patients might require more extended tip elevation than Caucasian ones.

The narrowest dorsal nasal bridge width is considered as a major landmark for the esthetic appearance of the nose, as it is positioned along the dorsal esthetic line and contributes majorly to the appearance of the frontal nose.[9] Considering that the nasal base was statistically larger in Asians than in Caucasians, it can be speculated based on the findings of this investigation that the nose of

Table 1
Overview of the study measurements and their respective definition and landmarks

Measurement	Definition/Landmarks
Face length (1)	Distance between Trichinion – Mentale
Face width (2)	Distance between Right Zygoma – Left Zygoma
Nasal length (3)	Distance between Glabella – Septum nasale
Nasal root width (4)	Distance between Right Eyebrow Margin – Left Eyebrow Margin
Dorsal bridge width (5)	Distance between Right Sellion – Left Sellion
Nasal base width (6)	Distance between Right Alar C – Left Alar C
Nasofrontal angle (7)	Angle between Glabella – Sellion and Sellion – Pronasion
Nasal dorsum angle (8)	Angle between Sellion – Rhinion and Rhinion – Pronasion
Nasolabial angle (9)	Angle between Columella – Nasal Septum and Nasal Septum – Upper lip
Glabella-nasion-sellion surface length (10)	Surface distance between the Glabella, Nasion, and Sellion
Dorsum surface length (11)	Surface distance between the Sellion, Supratip, and Pronasion

Asians appears rather triangular with a broad base (**Fig. 4**), whereas the nose of Caucasians, because of the broader dorsal bridge width and the smaller nasal base, appears rather trapezoid. Clinicians should consider this finding as a common injection point to ameliorate the nasolabial fold in the deep pyriform space.[10,11] By injecting into the deep pyriform space, the base of the nose also gains visual width, thus treating the nasolabial fold with this technique needs to be reconsidered on an individual basis to avoid further broadening of the nose in Asians. Inversely, broadening the nose of Caucasians might be desirable in some instances. Injecting into the deep pyriform space and optically widening the nasal base might be desirable. Regarding the dorsal bridge width, injectors should focus on Asians to define the dorsal esthetic line to produce sufficient results for the patient who do not only address dorsal hollowness and repositioning of the radix.

The presented results revealed that Caucasians displayed a greater dorsum surface length than Asians, which is remarkable, considering that the overall length of the nose in Asians was greater

Table 2
Mean values, standard deviation, and range for the investigated measurements of the entire study population (n = 160)

Measurement	Minimum	Maximum	Mean	Standard Deviation
Face length	166.78	219.17	189.61	10.36
Face width	89.24	153.30	122.78	8.47
Nasal length	58.65	83.62	69.48	5.34
Nasal root width	16.16	39.52	25.97	3.88
Dorsal bridge width	6.55	20.49	12.99	2.71
Nasal base width	24.16	43.49	33.62	4.17
Nasofrontal angle	126.66	161.39	144.94	5.92
Nasal dorsum angle	150.58	179.35	174.21	4.23
Nasolabial angle	94.44	143.39	117.02	10.23
Glabella-Nasion-Sellion surface length	8.74	32.60	18.70	4.28
Dorsum surface length	35.83	57.64	44.85	4.21

Table 3
Mean values and standard deviation for the investigated parameters in the male and female subpopulation of the Caucasian and Asian

	Caucasian		Asian	
	Male	Female	Male	Female
Face length	189.85 (9.49)	182.44 (9.26)	196.78 (9.64)	189.36 (8.08)
Face width	120.84 (5.92)	115.70 (6.35)	130.06 (7.81)	124.53 (6.69)
Nasal length	68.25 (4.29)	64.89 (3.34)	74.67 (3.94)	70.12 (4.50)
Nasal root width	25.49 (4.50)	26.59 (4.30)	26.19 (2.95)	25.64 (3.61)
Dorsal bridge width	15.29 (2.20)	14.05 (2.45)	12.05 (1.61)	10.60 (1.76)
Nasal base width	31.85 (2.41)	29.33 (3.00)	37.41 (2.91)	35.87 (2.48)
Nasofrontal angle	141.42 (5.45)	146.29 (6.26)	145.45 (5.25)	146.24 (5.23)
Nasal dorsum angle	174.07 (3.22)	175.55 (2.40)	174.74 (2.89)	172.56 (6.62)
Nasolabial angle	122.00 (8.65)	120.86 (10.27)	109.98 (9.04)	115.14 (8.44)
Glabella-Nasion-Sellion surface length	15.19 (2.42)	15.51 (2.21)	21.80 (2.21)	22.23 (3.64)
Dorsum surface length	47.79 (3.69)	43.69 (3.30)	46.78 (2.94)	41.12 (3.28)

than in Caucasians. The greater length of the dorsum of the nose, defined as the distance between the sellion and the pronasale, can be explained by a greater curvature of the Caucasian nose (quantitative, ie, not allowing conclusions on a convex or concave sloping of the dorsum). These findings are relevant to injectors as, especially in contouring the dorsum of the nose, greater quantities of fillers might be required for the augmentation of the dorsum of the nose in Caucasians than

in Asians. Greater injection volumes of soft-tissue fillers are related to a greater risk of injection-related complications such as skin necrosis or even blindness.[12,13] Injections to define the dorsum of the nose are performed by repositioning the radix of the nose from caudal to cranial.

The strengths of this study are the well-balanced and large sample size. To the knowledge of the authors, no previous investigations observed morphologic differences between Caucasians

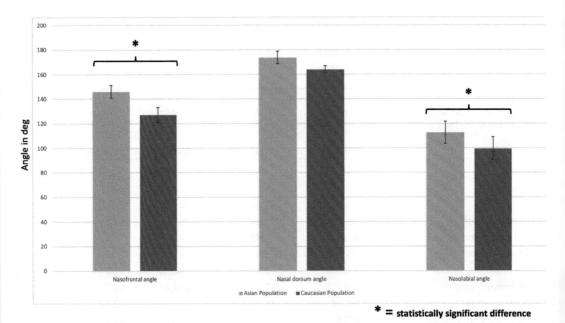

Fig. 4. Bar graph showing the mean values and standard deviation of the nasofrontal, nasal dorsum, and nasolabial angle in the lateral view of the nose. Asterisks (*) indicate a statistically significant difference between the Asian and Caucasian population.

and Asians in a sample size of n = 160 yet. Moreover, by using 3-dimensional surface imaging, the measurements are reproducible and objective and pose several advantages over classical anthropometric measurements performed on 2-dimensional photographs. All measurements were performed by the same investigator (Z.L.) to ensure consistency throughout the data acquisition. Although several previous investigations have focused on nasal morphometric differences between Asians and Caucasians, this study has tried to put the findings into a clinical context by linking them to potential implications when it comes to augmenting the nose using soft-tissue fillers.

A potential drawback of this investigation is the fact that even though 3-dimensional surface imaging is as close to depicting a real image of a subject as photographic technology allows; however, previous investigations have shown that measurement deviations can still not be eliminated.

SUMMARY

The results revealed an overall high number of statistically different measurements. Interestingly, the nose of Asians was statistically significantly longer than the nose of Caucasians, even when adjusted for facial height, the narrowest dorsal bridge width was statistically smaller in Asians than in Caucasians and the nasal base statistically larger, whereas the dorsal surface length was longer in Caucasians than in Asians. Injectors should be aware of these subtle differences between Caucasian and Asian noses during soft-tissue filler augmentations in the nasal region and use the presented findings as a guidance for potential pitfalls when injecting soft-tissue filler.

DISCLOSURE

The authors have nothing to disclose.

REFERENCES

1. The Aesthetic Society. Aesthetic Plastic Surgery National Databank Statistics. 2019:1-26.
2. Kassir R, Venkataram A, Malek A, et al. Non-Surgical Rhinoplasty: The Ascending Technique and a 14-Year Retrospective Study of 2130 Cases. Aesthetic Plast Surg 2020. https://doi.org/10.1007/s00266-020-02048-8.
3. Jung GS, Chu SG, Lee JW, et al. A Safer Non-surgical Filler Augmentation Rhinoplasty Based on the Anatomy of the Nose. Aesthetic Plast Surg 2019;43(2):447–52. https://doi.org/10.1007/s00266-018-1279-7.
4. Raggio BS, Asaria J. Filler Rhinoplasty. 2021 Jul 25. In: StatPearls [Internet]. Treasure Island (FL): StatPearls Publishing.
5. Kim NG, Park SW, Park HO, et al. Are differences in external noses between whites and Koreans caused by differences in the nasal septum? J Craniofac Surg 2015;26(3):922–6. https://doi.org/10.1097/SCS.0000000000001367.
6. Park J, Suhk J, Nguyen AH. Nasal Analysis and Anatomy: Anthropometric Proportional Assessment in Asians-Aesthetic Balance from Forehead to Chin, Part II. Semin Plast Surg 2015;29(4):226–31. https://doi.org/10.1055/s-0035-1564818.
7. Armijo BS, Brown M, Guyuron B. Defining the Ideal Nasolabial Angle. Plast Reconstr Surg 2012;129(3).
8. Gu Y, McNamara JA, Sigler LM, et al. Comparison of craniofacial characteristics of typical Chinese and Caucasian young adults. Eur J Orthod 2011;33(2):205–11. https://doi.org/10.1093/ejo/cjq054.
9. Mojallal A, Ouyang D, Saint-Cyr M, et al. Dorsal aesthetic lines in rhinoplasty: a quantitative outcome-based assessment of the component dorsal reduction technique. Plast Reconstr Surg 2011;128(1):280–8. https://doi.org/10.1097/PRS.0b013e318218fc2d.
10. Cotofana S, Gotkin RH, Frank K, et al. The Functional Anatomy of the Deep Facial Fat Compartments. Plast Reconstr Surg 2019;143(1):53–63. https://doi.org/10.1097/PRS.0000000000005080.
11. Surek CK, Vargo J, Lamb J. Deep Pyriform Space: Anatomical Clarifications and Clinical Implications. Plast Reconstr Surg 2016;138(1):59–64. https://doi.org/10.1097/PRS.0000000000002262.
12. Beleznay K, Carruthers JDA, Humphrey S, et al. Avoiding and treating blindness from fillers: A review of the world literature. Dermatol Surg 2015;41(10):1097–117. https://doi.org/10.1097/DSS.0000000000000486.
13. Beleznay K, Carruthers JDA, Humphrey S, et al. Update on Avoiding and Treating Blindness From Fillers: A Recent Review of the World Literature. Aesthet Surg J 2019. https://doi.org/10.1093/asj/sjz053.

Effect of Surgical versus Nonsurgical Rhinoplasty on Perception of the Patient
An Eye-Tracking-Based Investigation

Ramtin Kassir, MD[a], Sheila Kassir, MD[a], Luzi Hofmann[b], Nikita Breyer[b], Sebastian Cotofana, MD, PhD[c], Nicholas Moellhoff, MD[b], Michael G. Alfertshofer[b], Mia Cajkovsky[d], Konstantin Frank, MD[b,1], Lukas H. Kohler, MD[b,1,*]

KEYWORDS

• Rhinoplasty • Liquid rhinoplasty • Surgical rhinoplasty • Nasal anatomy

INTRODUCTION

The nose, because of its central location in the face, plays a major role in the appearance of a person (**Figs. 1–4**).[1–3] The shape and contour of a nose are defining characteristics of its beholder. Next to the periorbital region and the mouth, the gaze of a person predominantly dwells on the nasal region, from both frontal and lateral angles.[1,4,5] Especially in the lateral profile view, an unaesthetic nose can create an unaesthetic appearance of a person.[6,7] An imbalanced or unharmonious nose, either genetically determined or alternated by trauma, disease, or injury, can cause both psychological stress and an emotional burden to patients.[8–11] Moreover, the shape of a nose should be perceived not only from a purely aesthetic point of view but also from a functional one. Collapsed external or internal valves can cause breathing problems and consequently influence breathing physiology, which might lead to distress of the patient.[12,13]

Historically, open or closed rhinoplasty has been the only means to change the shape and contour of a nose; however, in the last decade the use of soft tissue fillers to alter the nasal region has significantly increased.[14] So-called liquid rhinoplasties have several advantages over classical surgical rhinoplasties. Short down times, short procedure times, ease of procedure, and lower costs for both the physician and the patient over surgical alteration of the nose have contributed to the spike of procedures in the last decade.[15–17] Notably, using soft tissue fillers to augment the nose does not allow one to perform sculpturing of the nose to the same extent as surgical rhinoplasty does, as only additive changes can be performed. This limits the degree of alteration and narrows the indication for liquid rhinoplasties.

A recent investigation by Frank and colleagues[18,19] has shown that duration of gaze is inversely correlated with aesthetic liking of facial features, whereas the time until fixation of a facial feature is positively correlated with aesthetic liking

Author disclosure: The authors declared no potential conflicts of interest with respect to the research, authorship, and publication of this article.
Funding: The authors received no financial support for the research, authorship, or publication of this article. The products used in this study were privately contributed by the first author for the purposes of this study.
[a] Park Avenue Plastic Surgery and Dermatology, Private Practice, New York City, NY, USA; [b] Division of Hand, Plastic and Aesthetic Surgery, University Hospital, LMU Munich, Munich 80336, Germany; [c] Department of Clinical Anatomy, Mayo Clinic College of Medicine and Science, Rochester, MN, USA; [d] Yuvell, Private Practice, Vienna, Austria
[1] Authors have contributed equally.
* Corresponding author. Division of Hand. Plastic and Aesthetic Surgery, University Hospital, LMU Munich, Pettenkoferstraße 8a, Munich 80336, Germany.
E-mail address: konstantin.frank@med.uni-muenchen.de

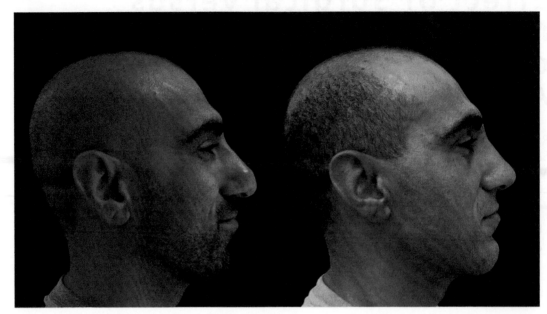

Fig. 1. Presurgical (*left*) and postsurgical (*right*) lateral photographs of a male patient that underwent surgical rhinoplasty.

of facial features. To date, the alteration of gaze when looking at preliquid and postliquid rhinoplasty images has not been investigated. Thus, the aim of this study is to investigate the extent of gaze deviation when looking at postliquid and surgical rhinoplasty images compared with the baseline images.

MATERIAL AND METHODS
Study Sample

This study investigated the eye movement pattern of 52 volunteers with a mean age of 32.0 ± 17.8 years, of which 28 were men and 24 were women. Volunteers were recruited at the

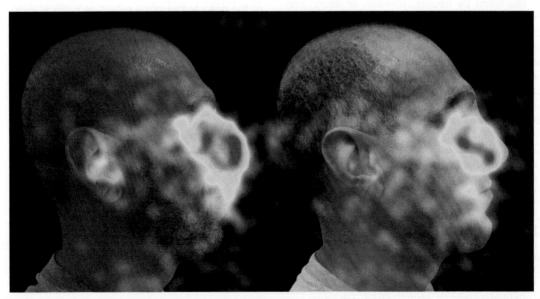

Fig. 2. Presurgical (*left*) and postsurgical (*right*) lateral photographs of a male patient that underwent surgical rhinoplasty with a superimposed heat map showing the average fixation of gaze. Note the higher intensity (*more reddish color*) in the nasal region in the preoperative image.

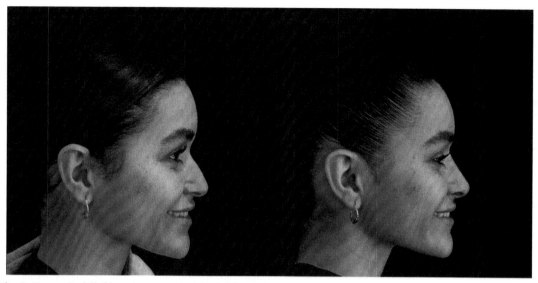

Fig. 3. Presurgical (*left*) and postsurgical (*right*) lateral photographs of a female patient that underwent liquid rhinoplasty.

Division of Hand, Plastic and Aesthetic Surgery, University Hospital, LMU Munich. All of the 52 recruited volunteers were laypersons.

Volunteers had to sign a consent form permitting the use of their demographic and result-related data for this study. The investigation was reviewed and approved by the Institutional Review Board of the LMU Munich (IRB protocol number: 20-1018). This study was conducted in accordance with regional laws (Germany) and good clinical practice.

Eye Movement Analyses

The eye movements were analyzed according to a previously published protocol with minor changes.[19] The gaze pattern of the included volunteers was recorded using a Tobii Pro Nano eye tracker (Tobii Pro AB, Stockholm, Sweden) with a frequency of 60 Hz. The eye tracker bar was connected and placed on top of a 15-in screen (339.5 mm × 244 mm) of a commercially available computer (Surface Laptop 3; Microsoft, Redmond,

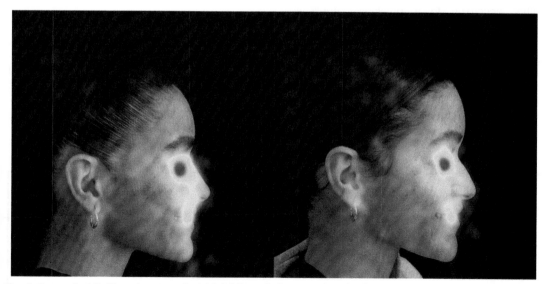

Fig. 4. Presurgical (*left*) and postsurgical (*right*) lateral photographs of a female patient that underwent liquid rhinoplasty with a superimposed heat map showing the average fixation of gaze. Note that there is barely a difference in the heat map upon visual inspection.

WA, USA). The defined area of eye capture and recording was 35 cm × 30 cm at a distance of 65 cm. The movement of the eyes was recorded as horizontal (x) and vertical (y) values over time of recording.

To allow for standardized conditions, all volunteers were shown the same set of visual stimuli in the same location, under almost identical light and seating conditions. Participants were required to sit upright on the same chair with a fixed backrest at a distance of 65 cm to the screen. Before presentation of the visual stimuli, a standardized 9-point calibration was performed to allow consistency throughout the eye movement analyses. If calibration was unsatisfying, it was performed until acceptable, as deemed by the investigator.

Visual Stimulus Presented

Photographs of a total of 6 different patients were presented to the participants. Each patient was shown in a perfectly frontal and perfectly (right) lateral view preoperatively and postoperatively, yielding a total of 24 images. Of those 6 patients, 3 patients underwent nonsurgical rhinoplasty and another 3 patients underwent surgical rhinoplasty. The images were displayed for a duration of 10 seconds. Between 2 displayed images a black screen was inserted for 2 seconds to allow some rest for the eyes. The presented visual stimuli were shown in a randomized sequence to avoid any bias. A stable eye fixation was defined as an eye fixation that was constant for a duration of at least 0.08 seconds. The rhinoplasties, both surgical and nonsurgical, were performed by the first author according to a previously published protocol.[14]

DATA ANALYSIS
Eye Movement Pattern Analysis

Data were analyzed according to a previously published protocol.[18,19] In brief, the following variables were captured:

- Time until first fixation in seconds of the nasal region (interval between initial display of the image and the first stable eye fixation)
- Time of fixation in seconds within the nasal region (duration of a stable eye fixation within the time of visual stimulus exposure = 10 seconds)
- Number of fixations within the nasal region

STATISTICAL ANALYSIS

The data were normally distributed, as assessed by Shapiro-Wilk's test ($P>.05$). Differences of the time until fixation, total time of fixation, and counts of fixation in the nasal region between preoperative and postoperative images were calculated using Student t test. All calculations were performed using SPSS Statistics 26 (IBM, Armonk, NY, USA), and results were considered statistically significant at a probability level of ≤ 0.05 to guide conclusions.

RESULTS
General Findings

Independent of surgical technique applied and view (lateral or frontal), the mean time until first fixation to the nasal region was 1.3 ± 1.9 seconds in the preoperative images and 1.45 ± 1.9 seconds in the postoperative images with $P = .292$. The mean time of total fixation was 1.67 ± 0.1 seconds in the preoperative images and 1.54 ± 0.1 seconds in the postoperative images with $P = .067$, whereas the number of fixations in the preoperative image was 4.32 ± 0.2 seconds and 4.13 ± 0.2 seconds in the postoperative image with $P = .232$.

Time Until Fixation

Mean time until first fixation did not differ significantly in the frontal or lateral view for both liquid rhinoplasties and surgical rhinoplasties when comparing gaze pattern for preoperative and postoperative images with $P \geq .135$. Further values are given in **Table 1**.

Table 1
Time to first fixation (mean value and standard deviation) of the nose from a frontal and lateral view, each after surgical and nonsurgical rhinoplasty, in seconds

Frontal				Lateral			
Nonsurgical		Surgical		Non Surgical		Surgical	
Pre operative	Post operative	Pre operative	Post operative	Pre operative	Post operative	Pre operative	Post operative
1.08 (1.7)	1.17 (1.5)	1.15 (1.7)	1.03 (1.4)	1.97 (2.3)	1.96 (2.3)	1.30 (1.8)	1.65 (2.0)

Total Time of Fixation

Total time of fixation only differed statistically significantly between the lateral preoperative and postoperative images of patients that underwent surgical rhinoplasty with 1.61 ± 1.6 seconds versus 1.23 ± 1.3 seconds ($P = .019$). In the frontal view of patients that underwent surgical rhinoplasty, time of fixation in the nasal region was 1.98 ± 1.8 seconds for the preoperative images and 2.06 ± 1.7 seconds for the postoperative images with $P = .677$. Further values are given in **Table 2**.

Count of Fixation

A statistically different number of counts of fixation in the nasal region was observed between the lateral preimages and postimages of patients that underwent surgical rhinoplasty with 4.78 ± 4.8 counts in the preoperative images and 3.81 ± 3.6 counts in the postoperative images with $P = .047$. No statistically significant differences of counts of fixation were observed in other images. Further values are given in **Table 3**.

DISCUSSION

This eye tracking-based investigation looked at differences between time until fixation of the nasal region, overall time of fixation within the nasal region, and number of counts within the nasal region of participants that looked for a predefined 10 seconds at frontal and lateral images of patients that underwent surgical and nonsurgical rhinoplasties. The results revealed that time until first fixation of the nasal region when looking at preoperative and postoperative images did not change for neither surgical nor nonsurgical rhinoplasties. However, overall time of fixation of the nasal region and number of fixations in the nasal region differed significantly for lateral images of patients that underwent surgical rhinoplasty.

The conducted study is not free of limitations. A limited amount of preoperative and postoperative images was shown to the volunteers, and a greater sample size might have revealed further findings; however, the authors have experienced that with increasing time of visual stimuli exposure attention decreases and the quality of eye tracking recording drops significantly. Thus, a total of 24 images were shown, yielding in a total stimulus presentation time of 4 minutes to avoid fatigue of the participants. The degree of deformation of the noses was different over the presented patients, which might have influenced the attention in the preoperative images owing to a greater variety of distraction. Moreover, visual stimuli presented were sole 2-dimensional photographs. Although standardized in terms of aperture, lighting, and capture time, 3-dimensional images might have given a better representation of the surgical outcome. Although randomization of the images was chosen to give an actual representation of real life, more distinct findings might have been revealed if the preoperative and postoperative images would have been juxtaposed. Moreover, no aesthetic rating of the outcomes was performed, which might have allowed one to draw further conclusions on the interplay between liking and gaze patterns.

A strength of this investigation is the age of participants, which was well distributed, including young and old subjects, giving an accurate representation of the population. Moreover, a standardized recording setting allowed one to limit biases as reflections on the screen or distraction by external influences. An additional strength of this investigation is its inherent novelty. Classically, postoperative outcomes are assessed using standardized and validated scales, like the GAIS (Global Aesthetic Improvement Scale) .[20–22] Using eye tracking technology to capture the gaze of people when looking at preoperative and postoperative images allows one to draw conclusions to which extent augmentations or changes to the nasal architecture can alter the perception of a person, from an objective point of view.

Interestingly, the time until first fixation did not differ significantly between the preoperative and

Table 2
Total fixation time (mean value and standard deviation) of the nose from a frontal and lateral view, each after surgical and nonsurgical rhinoplasty, in seconds

Frontal				Lateral			
Nonsurgical		Surgical		Nonsurgical		Surgical	
Pre operative	Post operative	Pre operative	Post operative	Pre operative	Post operative	Pre operative	Post operative
1.97 (1.8)	1.76 (1.6)	1.98 (1.8)	2.06 (1.7)	1.23 (1.4)	1.23 (1.4)	1.61 (1.6)	1.23 (1.3)

Table 3
Total number of fixations (mean and standard deviation) of the nose from a frontal and lateral view, each after surgical and nonsurgical rhinoplasty

Frontal				Lateral			
Nonsurgical		Surgical		Nonsurgical		Surgical	
Pre operative	Post operative	Pre operative	Post operative	Pre operative	Post operative	Pre operative	Post operative
6.11 (4.3)	5.66 (4.0)	5.60 (4.2)	6.35 (4.2)	3.68 (3.5)	3.80 (4.1)	4.78 (4.8)	3.81 (3.6)

postoperative images for neither surgical nor nonsurgical rhinoplasties. Previous studies have shown that aesthetic liking is strongly correlated to time until fixation and overall time of fixation of a region, that is, features that are considered aesthetic are fixated after a longer period of time than features that are considered unaesthetic, whereas the time of fixation is significantly shorter for features that are rated as pleasing than for features that are rated as unpleasing.[18,19] Assuming that the appearance of the nose was more pleasing after augmentation, the findings of this investigation are novel, as the focus/attention, that is, time until fixation of gaze, was not different in the preoperative and postoperative images. It was argued that the brain needs to process features that are unharmonious in a more precise way and tries to match the feature to the remaining face with more exertion once identified as nonapt. A reason for no statistical difference in time until fixation of the nasal region when looking at the presented frontal and lateral surgical and non surgical operative outcomes might be the randomized order. By the time the preoperative or the postoperative image was presented, the viewer might already have forgotten about the distracting or more harmonious appearance of the nose presented earlier.

However, considering that time of fixation has been shown to correlate inversely with aesthetic liking, the findings of this study are partially in line with previous literature. The nasal region was fixated for a significantly shorter time in the lateral view of surgical postoperative images, indicating that participants might have needed less time to put the appearance of the nose into context of the entire face. This might be attributable to the less unharmonious appearance. This study investigated count of fixations as an additional parameter, which has not been performed in previous investigations. The number of fixations in the nasal region was significantly shorter in the lateral images of postsurgical images than in presurgical images, furthermore strengthening the point that

less attention was paid to the nasal region, as it might have appeared more harmonious. Interestingly, no significant differences for time until fixation, overall time of fixation, and number of fixation counts were observed in the frontal view images. In all presented visual stimuli, the changes were more visible in the lateral view than in the frontal view. Surgeons should thus note and inform their patients that for cases similar to the presented ones, changes caused by surgical and nonsurgical rhinoplasty might appear more subtle in the frontal than in the lateral view.

Another important finding of this study is the fact that gaze, based on time until fixation, overall time of fixation, and number of fixation counts, was not significantly different in the preoperative and postoperative images of nonsurgical rhinoplasties. The changes performed did thus not alter the appearance of patients in a substantial way, when defining perception as gaze pattern. Although the presented cases have been reported to increase patient's quality of life and were reported as very satisfactory, surgeons might use this information to limit fear of patients that do not want to have an entirely altered appearance. To the educated and specialized observer, the changes in nose morphology are apparent; however, as the participants were all laypeople, it was not significantly apparent to viewers without a background in plastic surgery. Although fear of altered appearance might be reduced, physicians should, based on the findings of this study, also educate their patients that liquid rhinoplasties, although providing safe and fast results with little down time, might have less effect on the appearance of them compared with a surgical rhinoplasty. Whether a more profound change of appearance or rather subtle enhancement is desired by the patient needs to be elaborated during consultation.

SUMMARY

The results of this investigation suggest that the appearance of patients, especially in the lateral profile, is more profoundly altered when surgical rhinoplasty is performed, compared with nonsurgical rhinoplasty. Physicians should point this out to patients and find a tailored treatment plan for the patients that are seeking augmentation of the nasal region.

CLINICS CARE POINTS

The appearance of the nose, especially in the lateral view, has implications on the perception of the patientSurgical rhinoplasties change the appearance to a greater extent than nonsurgical rhinoplasties whether a more profound change of appearance or rather subtle enhancement is desired by the patient needs to be elaborated during consultation.

REFERENCES

1. Cai LZ, Kwong JW, Azad AD, et al. Where do we look? Assessing gaze patterns in cosmetic face-lift surgery with eye tracking technology. Plast Reconstr Surg 2019;144(1):63–70.
2. Dey JK, Ishii LE, Boahene KDO, et al. Measuring outcomes of Mohs defect reconstruction using eye-tracking technology. JAMA Facial Plast Surg 2019. https://doi.org/10.1001/jamafacial.2019.1072.
3. Frank K, Schuster L, Alfertshofer M, et al. How does wearing a facecover influence the eye movement pattern in times of COVID-19? Aesthet Surg J 2021. https://doi.org/10.1093/asj/sjab121.
4. Hessels RS. How does gaze to faces support face-to-face interaction? A review and perspective. Psychon Bull Rev 2020;27(5):856–81.
5. Frautschi RS, Dawlagala N, Klingemier EW, et al. The use of eye tracking technology in aesthetic surgery: analyzing changes in facial attention following surgery. Aesthet Surg J 2020;40(12):1269–79.
6. Jankowska A, Janiszewska-Olszowska J, Jedliński M, et al. Methods of analysis of the nasal profile: a systematic review with meta-analysis. Biomed Res Int 2021;2021:6680175.
7. Sarilita E, Rynn C, Mossey PA, et al. Nose profile morphology and accuracy study of nose profile estimation method in Scottish subadult and Indonesian adult populations. Int J Legal Med 2018;132(3):923–31.
8. Last U, Moses S, Mahler D. Mental health correlates of valid perception of nasal deformity in female applicants for aesthetic rhinoplasty. Aesthet Plast Surg 1983;7(2):77–80.
9. Hern J, Rowe-Jones J, Hinton A. Nasal deformity and interpersonal problems. Clin Otolaryngol Allied Sci 2003;28(2):121–4.
10. Sinno H, Izadpanah A, Thibaudeau S, et al. The impact of living with a functional and aesthetic nasal deformity after primary rhinoplasty: a utility outcomes score assessment. Ann Plast Surg 2012; 69(4):431–4.
11. Hern J, Hamann J, Tostevin P, et al. Assessing psychological morbidity in patients with nasal deformity using the CORE questionnaire. Clin Otolaryngol Allied Sci 2002;27(5):359–64.
12. Amodeo G, Scopelliti D. Nasal valve collapse: our treatment protocol. J Craniofac Surg 2017;28(4): e359–60.
13. Kalan A, Kenyon GS, Seemungal TA. Treatment of external nasal valve (alar rim) collapse with an alar strut. J Laryngol Otol 2001;115(10):788–91.
14. Kassir R, Venkataram A, Malek A, et al. Non-surgical rhinoplasty: the ascending technique and a 14-year retrospective study of 2130 cases. Aesthet Plast Surg 2020. https://doi.org/10.1007/s00266-020-02048-8.
15. Jung GS, Chu SG, Lee JW, et al. A safer non-surgical filler augmentation rhinoplasty based on the anatomy of the nose. Aesthet Plast Surg 2019; 43(2):447–52.
16. Lee W, Kim J-S, Oh W, et al. Nasal dorsum augmentation using soft tissue filler injection. J Cosmet Dermatol 2019;18. https://doi.org/10.1111/jocd.13018.
17. Rohrich RJ, Agrawal N, Avashia Y, et al. Safety in the use of fillers in nasal augmentation - the liquid rhinoplasty. Plast Reconstr Surg Glob Open 2020;8(8). https://doi.org/10.1097/GOX.0000000000002820.
18. Möllhoff N, Kandelhardt C, Ehrl D, et al. The impact of breast symmetry on eye movement and gaze pattern: an eye-tracking investigation. Aesthet Surg J 2021. https://doi.org/10.1093/asj/sjab285.
19. Frank K, Moellhoff N, Swift A, et al. In search of the most attractive lip-proportions and lip-volume – an eye tracking- and survey-based investigation. Plast Reconstr Surg. 2021; In Print.
20. Carruthers A, Carruthers J. A validated facial grading scale: the future of facial ageing measurement tools? J Cosmet Laser Ther 2010;12(5): 235–41.
21. Hernandez CA, Freytag DL, Gold MH, et al. Clinical validation of the temporal lifting technique using soft tissue fillers. J Cosmet Dermatol 2020. https://doi.org/10.1111/jocd.13621. jocd.13621.
22. Casabona G, Frank K, Koban KCKC, et al. Lifting vs volumizing-the difference in facial minimally invasive procedures when respecting the line of ligaments. J Cosmet Dermatol 2019;18(5). https://doi.org/10.1111/jocd.13089.

Superficial Nasal Filler Injections–How I do It

Arthur Swift, MD[a], Kent Remington, MD[b], Konstantin Frank, MD[c], Sebastian Cotofana, MD, PhD[d],*

KEYWORDS

- Non-surgical rhinoplasty • Profiloplasty • Soft tissue filler • Nasal anatomy
- Minimally invasive treatments

INTRODUCTION

Nasal enhancement is one of the most challenging and intriguing aesthetic procedures.[1–5] Although the nose is the most central and prominent facial feature, it should not be dominant while maintaining both a harmonious relationship with the face and its own intrinsic beauty.[6–9] In general, the contour and shape of the face, the skin's texture and thickness in the nasal region and balance and proportion with other facial features should be considered during the planning of minimally invasive injection therapy of the nose. The injector should always think in terms of improvement rather than perfection in these demanding cases. The apparent simplicity and falsely perceived ease of nonsurgical rhinoplasties using hyaluronic acid based soft tissue fillers (both by health care professionals and the public) associated with a short downtime and minimal discomfort have led to a significant increase in demand.[10] By addressing the 5 aesthetic components of the nose–the radix, the dorsum, the tip, the columella–alar complex, and the nasal base (**Fig. 1**)—facial appearance and attractiveness can be significantly improved and consequently influence the personal and psychological well-being of patients.[9,11–13] The anatomy of the nose is complex and the vast vascular network of the watershed vessels of the internal and external carotid system supplying the nose poses an increased risk for severe adverse events like skin necrosis or even blindness.[2,14] Beleznay and colleagues reported that more than half of all cases of blindness after soft tissue filler injections occurred after injections into the nose.[15,16] While aesthetic improvement of the nasal region is the main concern of many patients, precise deposition of hyaluronic acid into specific regions of the nose can also have significant influence on the physiology of the nose in terms of air flow during breathing. External valve dysfunction is a common issue and the bolstering of the collapsing tissue of the nose with soft tissue fillers can markedly improve air flow.[17–19] By structuring and supporting the nostril sill, air intake which is perhaps further compromised due to mucosal congestion and seasonal rhinitis can be improved at the nasal vestibule. Internal nasal valve collapse can occur with forced inspiration in congenitally narrow nasal airways, in elderly individuals with loss of overlying soft tissue and skin integrity due to age-related deterioration, or postoperatively after the loss of the scroll interlinking between upper and lower lateral cartilages as a result of the resection of the cephalic portion of the lower lateral cartilages during aesthetic rhinoplasty.[17,20] As for its internal valve analog, external nasal valve (alar rim) collapse can also be associated with any of the above as well as in genetically predisposed individuals with soft cartilages and thin skin.

Based on the vascular anatomy of the nose, as discussed in the following, the authors agree that injections are in general best performed in the

[a] Private Practice, Montreal, Quebec, Canada; [b] Remington Laser Dermatology Centre, Calgary, Canada; [c] Department for Hand, Plastic and Aesthetic Surgery, Ludwig – Maximilian University Munich, Germany; [d] Department of Clinical Anatomy, Mayo Clinic College of Medicine and Science, Mayo Clinic, Stabile Building 9-38, 200 First Street, Rochester, MN, 55905, USA

* Corresponding author.

E-mail address: cotofana.sebastian@mayo.edu

Facial Plast Surg Clin N Am 30 (2022) 183–191
https://doi.org/10.1016/j.fsc.2022.01.012

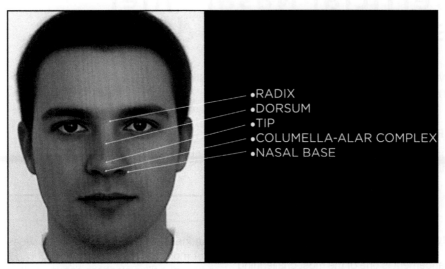

Fig. 1. Figure showing the 5 aesthetic components of the nose–the radix, the dorsum, the tip, the columella–alar complex, and the nasal base.

midline, targeting the supraperiosteal and supra-periochondrial layer. However, for some indications, especially off the midline of the nose, an intradermal injection technique needs to be performed to remain in the "safer" layer. It must be remembered there is no "safest" injection anywhere on the face, especially in the absence of ultrasound guidance, as all areas portend a certain risk of an adverse event. The nasal tip is particularly at risk whereby compression rather than intra-arterial deposition can lead to skin necrosis. In the following, the first author will share his experience regarding nasal filler injections performed superficially and incorporate patient assessment, anatomy of the nose, and injection techniques to provide guidance. The findings are the opinions of the authors and should be considered as such.

It should be stated from the outset that intradermal nasal injections must be approached with extreme caution in the postrhinoplasty patient and avoided in patients having undergone multiple previous operations due to the presence of both significant scarring and altered arterial and venous flow. The triad of a patient who lies about the number of previous operations, has a stern look from the outset of the consultation, and presents with a blunted nasal tip indicates an absolute contraindication to injection therapy.

ANATOMY OF THE NOSE

The nose is composed of both bony and cartilaginous structures, including the nasal bone with the ascending process of the maxilla; the upper lateral cartilages which are separated by the dorsal

septum; and the lower lateral cartilages which form in their medial aspect the domes and the medial crura, as well as the lateral crura in the lateral aspect. Lateral to the lower lateral cartilage, alar soft tissue can be found. The medial crura of the lower lateral cartilages become the footplates and are again separated in the midline by the caudal nasal septum, which connects to the anterior nasal spine of the maxilla.[21,22]

The mid–dorsum of the nose consists in general of 5 layers, while the radix and the tip do not possess a layered arrangement. In the mid–dorsum the five layers from superficial to deep are: (1) the skin envelope, (2) the subcutaneous areolar layer, (3) the vascular fibro–muscular layer, (4) the deep areolar layer, and (5) the perichondrium or periosteum.[23–25] (**Fig. 2**). The lack of a layered arrangement in the radix can be explained by the oblique course of the procerus muscle from its deep origin on the nasal bone to its superficial attachments in the glabella region. In the tip region, the lack of a layered arrangement can be explained by the fibrofatty nasal tissue.[14] The skin envelope of the nose varies in thickness with racial, gender, and ethnic disparities, and can be considered as one of the most sebaceous areas of the human body.[26]

Cranially, the nose receives its vascular supply from the dorsal nasal and the supratrochlear arteries, both terminal branches of the ophthalmic artery.[27,28] Caudally, the nose is supplied via the columellar arteries which branch off the superior labial branches of the angular arteries that also give off the lateral nasal arteries and the external nasal arteries. The lateral nasal, dorsal nasal, and

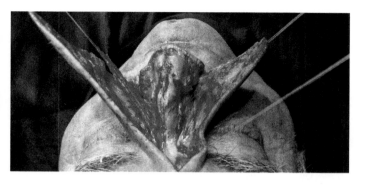

Fig. 2. Figure showing the layered arrangement of the nose: (1) the skin envelope, (2) the subcutaneous areolar layer, (3) the vascular fibro–muscular layer, (4) the deep areolar layer, and (5) the perichondrium or periosteum.

columellar arteries form a lobular plexus at the nasal tip.[29–32] As the dorsal nasal artery and supra-trochlear artery are terminal branches of the ophthalmic artery, most of the cases of blindness after soft tissue filler injections in the nose can be explained due to the retrograde flow of an inadvertent intraarterial injection of hyaluronic acid into the internal circulation. The subsequent occlusion of the central retinal artery leads to ischemia of the retina with varying degrees of visual impairment including total loss of visual perception of light.[33–35]

A recent ultrasound-based investigation of nasal anatomy revealed that the nasal soft tissue thickness from skin to bone/cartilage was on average 4.0 mm thick, thinnest at the mid–nasal dorsum with 3.39 mm, and thickest at the nasal radix with 4.38 mm. The arterial vasculature at the nasal radix was observed to course subdermally within the superficial fatty layer in most of the cases (**Fig. 3**); however, variations exist, and the vasculature was found in the supraperiosteal plane in 1.7% of patients. At the mid–nasal dorsum, the nasal vasculature was again located in most of the cases in the subdermal plane; however, in about 20%, the arteries were found in the supra-periosteal plane. Interestingly, at the nasal tip the nasal vasculature, similar to the nasal radix, was found in a significant majority in the subdermal layer while no vasculature was observed in any case in the supraperiochondrial plane. The vascular–fibromuscular layer is thin and can be considered as an attenuated aponeurosis. No muscle is present in this layer and loose fibrofatty areolar tissue can be observed in this plane.[14]

AGING OF THE NOSE

A main component of aging in the nasal region is bony resorption over adult life. Bony remodeling of the superomedial and inferolateral aspects of the orbital rim cause a flattening of the glabella and eyebrows, while the convexity of the upper forehead increases.[36] Furthermore, the pyriform aperture enlarges with increasing age and maxillary and pyriform recession increases.[37] This causes a widening of the alar base, drooping of the tip, and a more acute nasolabial angle with a resultant significant increase in both nasal length and soft tissue thickness.[14]

PATIENT ASSESSMENT AND AESTHETIC GOALS

To perform a proper nasal assessment, accepted concepts of a beautiful nose need to be revisited. Certainly, beauty lies in the eye of the beholder and an individual approach needs to be conducted for each patient. A key factor, however, in a beautifully perceived nose, probably resides in the proportion between nasal length, alar base width, intercanthal line to nasal tip, dorsal width, tip height, and intercanthal height. Put into numbers, the senior author judges that ideal nasal proportions resembling the golden ratio PHI (1.618) may be related to the intercanthal distance , that is,: intercanthal distance = 1.0, nasal length (lashline to columella) = 1.618, alar base width = 1.0, intercanthal line to nasal tip = 1.0, dorsal width = 0.618, and tip height = 0.618.[38] (**Fig. 4**)

Apart from spatial measurements, angles of the nose need to be respected. Exemplary, the nasofrontal angle at the radix, located at the lashline in women and at the supratarsal fold in Caucasian males, is considered to be aesthetically pleasing at around 130°.[39] Following the concept of nasal golden ratio proportions, the dorsum should be in general straight and no wider than phi (0.618) of the intercanthal distance, while in women the dorsum should lie 2 mm under a line drawn from the radix to the tip.[40](**Fig. 5A**). A beautiful nose should have 2 tip defining points (light reflexes) which are the most projecting aspects on the profile.[41] The tip location should be at the intercanthal distance from the intercanthal line to the tip projection, while the nasal length should be 1.618 times

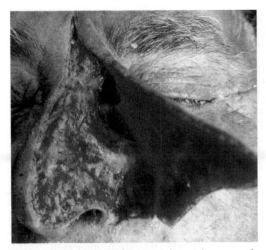

Fig. 3. Figure showing the arterial vasculature at the nasal radix to course subdermally within the superficial fatty layer.

the intercanthal distance from the radix to the columella. At the columella–alar complex, the nasolabial angle should be on average at around 95° to 115° in women (90°–95° in men) with a 2 to 3 mm show of the columella.[42] The nasal tip rotation should never give a turned up appearance to the nose, with a nasolabial angle of no more than 115° degrees, while at the base one should not be able to see more than just a hint of the nostril opening. The nasal base width should be in a vertical line with the inner canthus, that is, the intercanthal distance.[40] (**Fig. 5**B). Gender differences should be accounted for, as the masculine nose is characterized by a strong nasal dorsum in which there is a slight if any supratip break. In

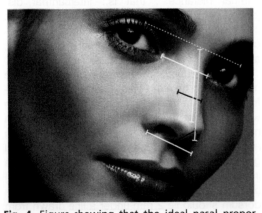

Fig. 4. Figure showing that the ideal nasal proportions might resemble the golden ratio PHI (1.618) related to the intercanthal distance that is,: intercanthal distance = 1.0; nasal length (lashline to columella) = 1.618; alar base width = 1.0; intercanthal line to nasal tip = 1.0; dorsal width = 0.618; tip height = 0.618.

men, unlike in women, there may be a little fullness laterally to the nasal bones at the rhinion.

INTRADERMAL DORSAL AUGMENTATION

Nasal dorsal augmentation is one of the most rewarding procedures in nasal injection therapy whereby a small amount of product can deliver an impressive result with a high degree of patient satisfaction. Injections of the dorsum are best performed on the periosteum (of the nasal bones) and or the perichondrium of the dorsal septum *in the midline* (relatively avascular plane) with either needle or cannula, and are commonly deployed in the radix area to soften the appearance of a dorsal hump. The senior author prefers a short bevel small gauge needle (eg, 31 g BDII at a 45° angle with the bevel down) versus a cannula whose port of entry is from the tip of the nose advanced cranially. This latter has difficulty hugging the periosteum due to the lack of defined layers at the nasal tip and due to the convexity of the dorsal hump. Before injection the BDII syringe is back loaded by removing and then replacing the plunger, maintaining sterility throughout.

Augmenting the radix extends the nasion cephalad and one should limit the location of this important angle to the eyelash line in the women to avoid masculinizing the appearance by creating the angle too high at the tarsal fold. Although supraperiosteal injections are preferable, superficial intradermal injections with minute amounts of product can also be done along the dorsum of the nose to correct asymmetries as well as irregularities apparent on both the profile and frontal view (**Fig. 6**). The result should always be checked from above the patient looking down from radix to tip to ensure that the dorsum displays a straight light reflex along the entire nasal length. The intradermal technique has proven especially useful in cases of difficult depressions or asymmetries located along the nasal vault sidewalls as well as the supratip region. The 31 g needle swathed onto the BDII syringe provides excellent control of product dispersion while maintaining the bevel of the needle facing down. Again, injections are conducted with miniboluses using the thenar eminence of the palm against the plunger to control product flow through a squeezing motion.

RESTORATION OF COLLAPSED EXTERNAL NASAL VALVES

The external nasal valve is made up of the septum, the medial and lateral crura of the lower lateral cartilage, and the premaxilla.[43,44] To strengthen the external nasal valve an intradermal injection of

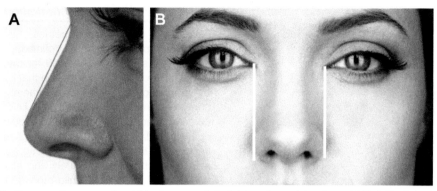

Fig. 5. Aesthetic appealing noses should be in general straight and no wider than phi (0.618) of the intercanthal distance, while in women the dorsum should lie 2 mm under a line drawn from the radix to the tip (A), while the nasal base width should be in a vertical line with the inner canthus, that is, the intercanthal distance (B).

soft tissue filler is performed using a 31 gauge 0.3 cc BDII syringe. The needle is inserted from lateral on a flat plane between the leaves of skin caudal to the inferior edge of the lower lateral cartilage (**Fig. 7**). The small syringe and needle allow for controlled deposition of minute boluses of 0.01 cc to be injected intradermally and antegrade, avoiding the more medial beautiful soft triangle facet. Slight pressure is applied to the plunger all the while observing the color of the overlying skin which will temporarily blanch due to pressure. This injection is also efficacious at correcting a retracted nostril seen as a stigmatizing complication of rhinoplasty performed with endonasal incisions (**Fig. 8**). For the treatment of collapsed external nasal valves,

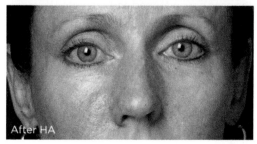

Before

After HA

Fig. 6. Figure showing the frontal view of a woman before and after superficial intradermal injections with minute amounts of product along the dorsum of the nose to correct asymmetries.

further intradermal nasal sill injections can be performed from medial to lateral toward the alar base, aiming for the ipsilateral lateral canthus (**Fig. 9**). Again it must be emphasized that the use of a short 31 g needle allows precise positioning of the product while a shallow injection angle should be kept at all times. Gentle massage is crucial to layer the product in the dermal plane and relieve the pressure on the overlying skin. Once completed, the patient is asked to forcefully inhale to assess the correction and necessity of further injection. Typical volume is less than 0.15 cc of an intermediate G′ product for all areas of the external valve treated. Again it is of uttermost importance to inject slowly, constantly watching for blanching of the skin which will occur temporarily at the alar rim in most cases due to the compression of the overlying skin. All nasal injection patients remain in the clinic for 15-minutes posttreatment to confirm the return of normal perfusion and capillary refill to the treated area. In the rare event of persistent blanching after 15 minutes, reversal of injected product is accomplished with hyaluronidase.

RESTORATION OF COLLAPSED INTERNAL NASAL VALVES

The internal nasal valve area is made up by the nasal septum medially, the floor of the nose inferiorly, the upper lateral cartilage and its scroll interdigitation with the lower lateral cartilage laterally, and the head of the inferior turbinate superiorly and laterally.[45] Similar to injections into the external nasal valve, intradermal injections with a backloaded 31 g 0.3 cc BDII syringe are performed into the collapsing skin overlying the internal nasal valve area with minute boluses of 0.01 cc (in a shallow injection angle) to provide structure and support. This in effect can be likened to creating a suspension bridge preventing the collapse of

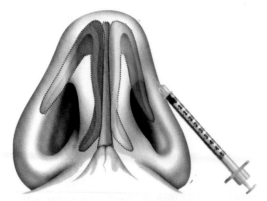

Fig. 7. Figure showing the insertion of the needle from lateral on a flat plane between the leaves of skin caudal to the inferior edge of the lower lateral cartilage.

the skin with the negative pressure generated during inspiration. If internal valve collapse persists on forceful inspiration, further injection boluses may need to be applied. It is important not to inject subdermally as product below the skin may not only contribute to underlying cartilage invagination (worsening the obstruction) but also in order to avoid the vasculature at this deeper depth.

CORRECTION OF COLUMELLAR SHOW

Another indication for intradermal injection of soft tissue filler in the nasal region is the correction of minimal or excessive columellar show. A retracted columella can be corrected using a combination of supraperiosteal (on the nasal spine) and intradermal injections of soft tissue filler to increase the columellar show to about 2 to 3 mm. The paired columellar arteries reside in the subdermal plane and injections at this level are to be avoided. On the contrary, excessive columellar show due to retracted alar rims can be reduced by intradermal injection into the alar rim as outlined above. The same precautions of observing the injected skin and gentle massaging are paramount to avoiding adverse complications.

Increasing Tip Height and Definition

Correction of tip asymmetries, as well as increasing projection and definition, are techniques that should be reserved for the seasoned injector. The nasal tip is unique in that it is supplied by a myriad of end arteries whereby external compression can actually lead to clinically significant impaired blood flow and subsequent skin necrosis, similar to a pressure ulcer. Any minute intradermal injections to correct tip asymmetries must be performed delicately and slowly with a low G′ product, all the while monitoring the skin for evidence of vascular compromise. Any blanching observed during injection must be immediately massaged to soften compressive effects and the skin checked for an appropriate capillary refill. The intradermal layer should never be targeted for more copious injections in an attempt to increase tip projection. A safer route would be to "underpin" the tripod responsible for supporting the tip by injecting on the periosteum of the nasal spine and the pyriform fossae with a high G′ product. Further augmentation of tip height can then be achieved by using a drop technique of the tip onto the BDII needle from the midline of the columella, targeting the relatively avascular area between the medial crura. Slow injection of a moderate G′ product is then performed while the fingers of the free hand create a barrier to uncontrolled spread. Typical volume does not exceed 0.2 cc of hyaluronic acid.

DISCUSSION

Nasal injections, while highly rewarding and portending a high satisfaction rate, are the most precarious procedures in soft tissue facial enhancement. Due to the complex vascular interplay, the proximity to several anastomoses of the internal and external circulatory system, and lack of precise layering in certain areas of the nose, vascular compromise is at higher risk when augmenting the nose. While in general deep injections in the nose are performed and supported by recent studies that investigated the vascular arrangement

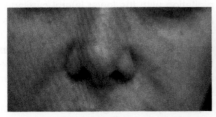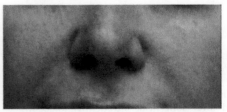

Fig. 8. Figure showing the frontal view of a woman before and after correcting a retracted nostril seen as a stigmatizing complication of rhinoplasty performed with endonasal incisions.

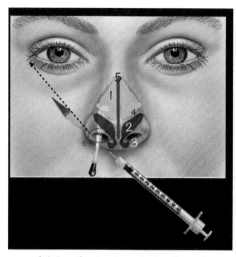

1 Upper lateral cartilage

2 Lower lateral cartilage

3 Nasal Sill

4 Internal Valve

5 Nasal Septum

6 External Valve

Fig. 9. Figure explaining the treatment of collapsed external nasal valves.

of the nose, the presented techniques inject product in the intradermal layer for specific indications.[14]

While it seems counterintuitive to inject intradermally in a region that lacks a layered arrangement, several precautions are used during the injection procedure to minimize vascular compromise. Recent investigations have shown that the spread of product depends on the size of the needle that is used for injection, the rheology of the product, and on the injection angle with which the product is injected. A higher needle diameter correlates significantly with product spread, while a higher injection angle concomitantly increases migration of product along cannula or needle channels. By choosing a shallow injection angle and using a very small needle (31 g), spread of product is limited with the presented injection technique. Furthermore, a correlation between bolus volume of injected product and risk of vascular compromise has been established in the literature. By injecting minute units of filler (0.01 cc) and continual monitoring for blanching of the skin, vascular compromise and the risk of permanent damage to the microcirculation of the overlying soft tissue is minimized. Proper product choice is essential for intradermal injections in the nasal region, as a balance in terms of the viscoelastic properties necessary for example, to support the collapsed valve while avoiding excessive pressure on the microcirculation is necessary.[46–48]

SUMMARY

Intradermal injections of the nose to ameliorate internal and external valve collapse, to create appropriate columellar show, or to improve nasal contours is a demanding yet rewarding procedure for patient and physician. It forms an integral part of the experienced injector's minimally invasive armamentarium in enhancing facial attractiveness, whereby a small difference in anatomy makes a big difference in appearance. The authors in no way imply that noninvasive injection therapy should replace definitive surgical rhinoplasty, which still remains the gold standard for nasal enhancement. In fact, nasal injection therapy has proven to be an important adjunct to occasional postrhinoplasty minor corrections in the senior author's plastic surgical practice.

As with all facial injections, precise knowledge of anatomy and applied techniques are essential to minimize adverse events. Injectors should always be aware that the nose is one of the riskiest areas of the face to inject, due to its complex anatomy and its vascular proximity to the neighboring orbit.

DISCLOSURE

The authors declared no potential conflicts of interest with respect to the research, authorship, and publication of this article.

FUNDING

The authors received no financial support for the research, authorship, or publication of this article. The products used in this study were privately contributed by the authors of this study.

REFERENCES

1. Humphrey CD, Arkins JP, Dayan SH. Soft tissue fillers in the nose. Aesthet Surg J 2009;29(6): 477–84.
2. Tansatit T, Moon H-J, Rungsawang C, et al. Safe planes for injection rhinoplasty: a histological

analysis of midline longitudinal sections of the asian nose. Aesthetic Plast Surg 2016;40(2):236–44.

3. Kurkjian TJ, Ahmad J, Rohrich RJ. Soft-tissue fillers in rhinoplasty. Plast Reconstr Surg 2014;133(2):121e–6e.

4. Lee W, Kim J-S, Oh W, et al. Nasal dorsum augmentation using soft tissue filler injection. J Cosmet Dermatol 2019;18. https://doi.org/10.1111/jocd.13018.

5. Lee W, Koh I-S, Oh W, et al. Ocular complications of soft tissue filler injections: a review of literature. J Cosmet Dermatol 2020;19(4):772–81.

6. Greer SE, Matarasso A, Wallach SG, et al. Importance of the nasal-to-cervical relationship to the profile in rhinoplasty surgery. Plast Reconstr Surg 2001;108(2):522–5.

7. Leong SC, Eccles R. A systematic review of the nasal index and the significance of the shape and size of the nose in rhinology. Clin Otolaryngol 2009;34(3):191–8.

8. Bhatia AF. Facial profile-esthetics and acceptance. Indian J Dent Res 1989;1(2–3):45–53.

9. Pearson DC, Adamson PA. The ideal nasal profile: rhinoplasty patients vs the general public. Arch Facial Plast Surg 2004;6(4):257–62. https://doi.org/10.1001/archfaci.6.4.257.

10. ASPS National CLearinghouse of Plastic Surgery Procedural Statistics. Plastic Surgery statistics report 2019. Published online 2019:1-25. Available at: https://www.plasticsurgery.org/documents/News/Statistics/2019/plastic-surgery-statistics-full-report-2019.pdf.

11. Di Rosa L, Cerulli G, De Pasquale A. Psychological Analysis of non-surgical rhinoplasty. Aesthet Plast Surg 2020;44(1):131–8.

12. Springer IN, Zernial O, Warnke PH, et al. Nasal shape and gender of the observer: implications for rhinoplasty. J Craniomaxillofac Surg 2009;37(1):3–7.

13. Herruer JM, Prins JB, van Heerbeek N, et al. Does self-consciousness of appearance influence postoperative satisfaction in rhinoplasty? J Plast Reconstr Aesthet Surg 2018;71(1):79–84.

14. Alfertshofer MG, Frank K, Ehrl D, et al. The layered anatomy of the nose: an ultrasound-based investigation. Aesthet Surg J 2021. https://doi.org/10.1093/asj/sjab310.

15. Beleznay K, Carruthers JDA, Humphrey S, et al. Avoiding and treating blindness from fillers. Dermatol Surg 2015;41(10):1097–117.

16. Beleznay K, Carruthers JDA, Humphrey S, et al. Update on avoiding and treating blindness from fillers: a recent review of the world literature. Aesthet Surg J 2019;39(6):662–74.

17. Amodeo G, Scopelliti D. Nasal valve collapse: our treatment protocol. J Craniofac Surg 2017;28(4):e359–60.

18. Deroee AF, Younes AA, Friedman O. External nasal valve collapse repair: the limited alar-facial stab approach. Laryngoscope 2011;121(3):474–9.

19. Riechelmann H, Karow E, DiDio D, et al. External nasal valve collapse - a case-control and interventional study employing a novel internal nasal dilator (Nasanita). Rhinology 2010;48(2):183–8.

20. Wittkopf M, Wittkopf J, Ries WR. The diagnosis and treatment of nasal valve collapse. Curr Opin Otolaryngol Head Neck Surg 2008;16(1):10–3.

21. Patel RG. Nasal anatomy and function. Facial Plast Surg 2017;33(1):3–8.

22. Oneal RM, Beil RJ. Surgical anatomy of the nose. Clin Plast Surg 2010;37(2):191–211.

23. Anderson KJ, Henneberg M, Norris RM. Anatomy of the nasal profile. J Anat 2008;213(2):210–6.

24. Jung GS, Chu SG, Lee JW, et al. A safer non-surgical filler augmentation rhinoplasty based on the anatomy of the nose. Aesthet Plast Surg 2019;43(2):447–52.

25. Kim TK, Jeong JY. Surgical anatomy for Asian rhinoplasty. Arch Craniofac Surg 2019;20(3):147–57.

26. Cho GS, Kim JH, Yeo N-K, et al. Nasal skin thickness measured using computed tomography and its effect on tip surgery outcomes. Otolaryngol Head Neck Surg 2011;144(4):522–7.

27. Choi DY, Bae JH, Youn KH, et al. Topography of the dorsal nasal artery and its clinical implications for augmentation of the dorsum of the nose. J Cosmet Dermatol 2018;17(4):637–42.

28. Agorgianitis L, Panagouli E, Tsakotos G, et al. The supratrochlear artery revisited : an anatomic review in favor of modern cosmetic applications in the area 2020;1(2):1–6.

29. Rohrich RJ, Gunter JP, Friedman RM. Nasal tip blood supply: an anatomic study validating the safety of the transcolumellar incision in rhinoplasty. Plast Reconstr Surg 1995;95(5):791–5.

30. Toriumi DM, Mueller RA, Grosch T, et al. Vascular anatomy of the nose and the external rhinoplasty approach. Arch Otolaryngol Head Neck Surg 1996;122(1):24–34.

31. Bravo BSF, Bravo LG, Mariano Da Rocha C, et al. Evaluation and proportion in nasal filling with hyaluronic acid. J Clin Aesthet Dermatol 2018;11(4):36–40.

32. Jung DH, Kim HJ, Koh KS, et al. Arterial supply of the nasal tip in Asians. Laryngoscope 2000;110(2 Pt 1):308–11.

33. Townshend A. Blindness After Facial Injection. J Clin Aesthet Dermatol 2016;9(12):E5–7. http://www.ncbi.nlm.nih.gov/pubmed/28210400.

34. Kim SN, Byun DS, Park JH, et al. Panophthalmoplegia and vision loss after cosmetic nasal dorsum injection. J Clin Neurosci 2014;21(4):678–80.

35. Loh KTD, Chua JJ, Lee HM, et al. Prevention and management of vision loss relating to facial filler injections. Singapore Med J 2016;57(8):438–43.

36. Frank K, Gotkin RH, Pavicic T, et al. Age and gender differences of the frontal bone: a computed tomographic (CT)-based study. Aesthet Surg J 2018. https://doi.org/10.1093/asj/sjy270.

37. Cotofana S, Gotkin RH, Morozov SP, et al. The relationship between bone remodeling and the clockwise rotation of the facial skeleton. Plast Reconstr Surg 2018. https://doi.org/10.1097/prs.0000000000004976.

38. Bueller H. Ideal facial relationships and goals. Facial Plastic Surgery 2018;34(5):458–65.

39. Naini FB, Cobourne MT, Garagiola U, et al. Nasofrontal angle and nasal dorsal aesthetics: a quantitative investigation of idealized and normative values. Facial Plast Surg 2016;32(4):444–51.

40. Brito ÍM, Avashia Y, Rohrich RJ. Evidence-based Nasal Analysis for Rhinoplasty: the 10-7-5 Method. Plast Reconstr Surgery Glob Open 2020;8(2):e2632.

41. Park SS. Fundamental principles in aesthetic rhinoplasty. Clin Exp Otorhinolaryngol 2011;4(2):55–66.

42. Pearlman SJ. Surgical treatment of the nasolabial angle in balanced rhinoplasty. Facial Plast Surg 2006;22(01):28–35.

43. Hamilton GS 3rd. The external nasal valve. Facial Plast Surg Clin North Am 2017;25(2):179–94.

44. Tasca I, Ceroni Compadretti G, Sorace F. Nasal valve surgery. Acta Otorhinolaryngol Ital 2013;33(3):196–201.

45. Sulsenti G, Palma P. [The nasal valve area: structure, function, clinical aspects and treatment. Sulsenti's technic for correction of valve deformities]. Acta Otorhinolaryngol Ital 1989;9(Suppl 22):1–25.

46. Pavicic T, Mohmand HM, Yankova M, et al. Influence of needle size and injection angle on the distribution pattern of facial soft tissue fillers. J Cosmet Dermatol 2019. https://doi.org/10.1111/jocd.13066.

47. Pavicic T, Yankova M, Schenck TL, et al. Subperiosteal injections during facial soft tissue filler injections-Is it possible? J Cosmet Dermatol 2019. https://doi.org/10.1111/jocd.13073.

48. Rosamilia G, Hamade H, Freytag DL, et al. Soft tissue distribution pattern of facial soft tissue fillers with different viscoelastic properties. J Cosmet Dermatol 2020;19(2):312–20.

The Deep Columellar Approach for Liquid Rhinoplasty – A Case Series of 511 Procedures over 16 years

Fabiano Nadson Magacho-Vieira, MD[a,b,*], Michael G. Alfertshofer[c], Sebastian Cotofana, MD, PhD[d]

KEYWORDS

- Liquid rhinoplasty • Non-surgical rhinoplasty • Filler • Nose • Safety • Case series

KEY POINTS

- A growing number of cadaveric and ultrasonographic studies demonstrate that injecting the nose accurately in the supraperiosteal or supraperichondrial layers can significantly reduce the risk of vascular complications related to soft-tissue fillers.
- Blunt cannulas are suggested in high-risk regions in an attempt to reduce vessel injury, but precisely positioning them in the specific, supraperiosteal or supraperichondrial, layers of the nose can be challenging.
- Using a deep columellar approach to the tip and the cartilaginous dorsum and a lateral approach to the bony dorsum allows the injector to accurately identify the submuscular plane and double-check the cannula placement in the desired layer before filler injection.
- The low rate of 2.74% and the low severity of reported adverse events can be drawn back to the precise and verifiable soft-tissue filler placement in the deep fatty layers (supraperiosteal and supraperichondrial), using blunt cannulas.

 Video content accompanies this article at http://www.facialplastic.theclinics.com.

INTRODUCTION

The surface anatomy of the nose is determined by a complex system of angles, prominences, and contours that are relatively consistent among individuals. A nasal profile view that seems straight or slightly concave, for example, yields significantly more satisfaction with appearance than one that presents nasal humps, irrespective of the subject's gender.[1] A wide range of operations that were designed to achieve that beauty ideal have been the subject of innumerable publications.[2–4]

Rhinoplasty is a highly complex and intricate surgery, with an overabundance of opportunities

Author disclosure: Dr F.N. Magacho-Vieira is a regular speaker and participates in advisory boards for Galderma.

Funding: The authors received no financial support for the research, authorship, and publication of this article.

[a] Electrophysiology Laboratory, Ceara State University, Avenida Dr. Silas Munguba, 1700, Fortaleza, CE, Brazil 60714-903; [b] Department of Clinical, Aesthetic and Surgical Dermatology, Batista Memorial Hospital, Rua Professor Dias da Rocha, 1530, 6o. Andar, Fortaleza, CE, Brazil 60170-311; [c] Department of Hand, Plastic and Aesthetic Surgery, Ludwig-Maximilians-University, Geschwister-Scholl-Platz 1, Munich, Germany 80539; [d] Department of Clinical Anatomy, Mayo Clinic College of Medicine and Science, 200 1st St SW, Rochester, MN 55905, USA

* Corresponding author. Clinica Magacho – Avenida Desembargador Moreira, 1300, Sala 1419 - Torre Norte – Fortaleza, Ceará, Brasil, 60170-002.

E-mail address: dr.fabiano@clinicamagacho.com.br

Facial Plast Surg Clin N Am 30 (2022) 193–203
https://doi.org/10.1016/j.fsc.2022.01.005
1064-7406/22/© 2022 Elsevier Inc. All rights reserved.

for errors that can lead to complications.[5] There is always the possibility of prolonged downtime, with postoperative edema and bruising, apart from other adverse results, such as iatrogenic deformities, even as a late presentation.[6] Therefore, a number of individuals are not willing to undergo surgical intervention.

The terms "liquid rhinoplasty" or "nonsurgical rhinoplasty" (NSR) have been frequently used to refer to the use of soft-tissue fillers to mitigate aesthetic deformities of the nasal sidewalls and dorsum, to lengthen a short nose, and/or to alter the nasolabial angle affecting tip projection or rotation.[7–9] While it may not be considered a substitute for surgery, bearing a more restricted range of indications, the injection of autologous or heterologous fillers is minimally invasive and can potentially help patients who are concerned about financial expenses, anesthetic risk or downtime.[10] The first modern publications on the subject date from the mid-1980s, but nonsurgical options are increasingly more popular today, with the advent of several new synthetic injectable fillers with different rheological characteristics.[9]

Although, in general, dermal fillers can be considered safe, adverse reactions still may arise. Those include immunoreactions, infections, and granulomas, along with more severe and devastating complications, such as skin necrosis or blindness due to retinal artery occlusion.[11,12] Given the complexity and variability of nasal vascularization, reports of adverse effects of liquid rhinoplasty have been described over the years.[13–17] It is, in fact, essential to know and document possible complications related to the different techniques, as well as to estimate a safety level for future treatments.

The keys to safety in NSR can be referred to as maintaining the midline of the nose during cannula advancement, the use of blunt cannulas, and precise, low pressure, low volume, filler injection into the deep layers (supraperiosteal or supraperichondrial). This study describes a 4-step treatment algorithm that intends to meet those directives, following a standardized and reproducible methodology. It also reviews and documents treatments performed with this approach over more than 16 years, focusing on vascular complications.

MATERIAL AND METHODS
Study Setup

This retrospective study collected and analyzed secondary data from the medical records of patients who underwent liquid rhinoplasty at the dermatology outpatient clinic of the Batista Memorial Hospital, located in Fortaleza, Brazil between September 2004 and March 2021. Procedures were performed by or under the supervision of the first author (F.M.), using the 4-step injection algorithm including the deep columellar approach described in this publication.

Data collected for this study were: initials, gender, age, date, prior surgical rhinoplasty history, filler used, and areas treated for each liquid rhinoplasty procedure. Occurrence, diagnostic, and treatment of adverse effects possibly related to the NSR and reported by the assisting physician, were also documented. The anonymity and data security of patients was preserved at all times. Medical records with incomplete, illegible, or inaccessible data were excluded.

All methods and resources were performed in accordance with good clinical practice and institutional and national ethics standards as well as with Brazilian regulations and laws. Ethical approval for the retrospective clinical study was granted by the assigned research ethics committee (Paulo Picanço College; CAAE 33791720.1.0000.9267).

Study Sample

Patients were selected for undergoing liquid rhinoplasty after meeting the following criteria: (1) subjective patient dissatisfaction with nose profile; (2) unwillingness to undergo surgical rhinoplasty in the near future; (3) no active autoimmune disease or history of soft-tissue related autoimmune diseases; and (4) no other contraindications for filler injection or preexisting condition that could impact the patients' safety.

A visual analysis of the nose is usually sufficient to determine whether or not to accept the patient's complaint as realistic and combine patient preferences with surgical or nonsurgical options.[18] We recommend a quick 10-point checklist to determine a good prognosis for NSR (**Box 1**).

Pretreatment Examination

All patients undergo an appointment prior to the procedure to take pretreatment photographs and discuss the intervention, posttreatment care, and possible complications, as well as to set realistic expectations. The facial skin is visually analyzed for infections or other contraindications. The patient is queried about their health history and previous surgical procedures. The nasal vestibule and cavity are evaluated for signs of obstruction or inflammation. Subjects with excessive columellar show were informed about possible worsening of that characteristic after filler injection in the columellar area.

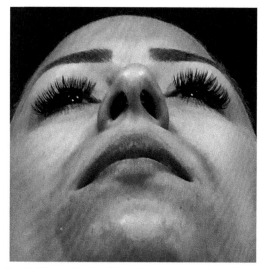

Fig. 1. Photograph of female patient's nose and nostrils format.

Photographic Documentation

Standard frontal, 45° lateral, and nose profile photos are mandatory. We also suggest the documentation of the nostrils format, positioning the camera distal to the chin (**Fig. 1**). Lighting from above can further evidence nasal irregularities or deviations.[19]

Injection Technique

The procedure consists of a 4-step injection technique, whereby each step is intended to correct or "beautify" key angles (**Fig. 2**) and corresponding anatomic structures (**Table 1**). Two cannula insertion (entry) points are used (Video 1):

1. A caudal cannula insertion point is used to treat the midline of the tip and the whole cartilaginous nasal dorsum. The nondominant hand (NDH) is used to create a "tent" on the philtrum by lifting the columella, and the midline on the base of that "tent" is marked, approximately 5 mm caudal to the columellar-labial junction (**Fig. 3**), to prevent filler backflow through the puncture.
2. A lateral cannula entry point is used to correct the nasofrontal angle when needed. The cannula is inserted in the lateral nasal dorsum, aligned to the deepest point of the patient's nasofrontal angle (= nose radix) (**Fig. 4**). The NDH

is used to evidence the bone and the point is marked.

Step 1 – the Anterior Nasal Spine

Using the caudal cannula insertion site (philtrum entry point) and holding the columella with the NDH, a 22G cannula is inserted through the skin and directed to the anterior nasal spine, until it reaches the fibromuscular layer (= nasal superficial musculoaponeurotic system[20]).

As the NDH moves the columella away from the bone (**Fig. 5**), the injector should feel a "jolt" when

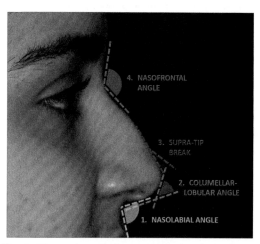

Fig. 2. Illustration of the supra-tip break (*red*) and other angles in the nose contouring in a profile photograph. The ideal nasolabial angle (*green*) is approximately 90° to 110°, the columellar-lobular angle (*orange*) is approximately 30° to 45°, the nasofrontal angle (*blue*) is approximately 115° to 135°.

Table 1
Liquid Rhinoplasty procedure steps and related anatomic structures and profile angles on the nose

	Related Anatomic Structure	Related Nose Profile Angle
STEP 1	Anterior Nasal Spine	Nasolabial Angle
STEP 2	Columella	Columellar-lobular Angle
STEP 3	Tip and/or Supra-tip	Columellar-lobular Angle Supra-tip Break
STEP 4	Radix	Nasofrontal Angle

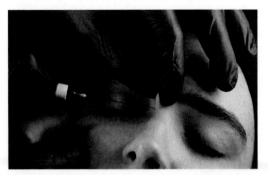

Fig. 4. Correction of the nasofrontal angle with the use of a cannula insertion in the lateral nasal dorsum, aiming at the deepest point of the nasofrontal angle.

the cannula pierces the muscle. The NDH should now hold the septum and feel the anterior nasal spine, so the cannula can touch the bone precisely in the midline, in the space between the posterior septal angle and the anterior nasal spine (approximately 5 mm large[21]). A bolus of 0.1 up to 0.3 mL of the filler is slowly injected (Video 2).

The desired submuscular layer is verified by moving the nasal septum back and forth, away from the nasal spine (the cannula must not move), confirming the cannula is, in fact, piercing the muscle (Video 3).

Using a philtral entry point simplifies the positioning of the filler under the feet of the medial crura of the lower lateral cartilages, as injectors must be careful to always direct the cannula toward the columellar-labial junction and not to the base of the anterior nasal spine, so that the volume provided by the filler affects mostly the columellar base and minimally the upper lip.

Step 2 – the Columella

For the second step, the NDH, still holding the base of the columella, makes a "lever" movement

(**Fig. 6**A), creating a "tent" in the philtrum region (**Fig. 6**B). The cannula is slightly retracted from the previous injection point and, without leaving the submuscular layer, is then directed parallel to the columella and advanced until it reaches a line that connects the highest point of the nostrils (columella-lobular junction), preserving the infra-tip from filler injection (**Fig. 7**). The tip of the cannula might be easily palpated on this limiting line or on the lateral walls of the nasal septum. Approximately 0.1 to 0.3 mL of the filler are then injected in a retrograde manner, down to the columellar-labial junction (Video 4). The injection is interrupted, the cannula is removed, and we proceed to Step 3.

Step 3 – the Tip and Supra-Tip

Still using the philtrum access point and the same "lever" or "crowbar" movement described in Step 2, the cannula is carefully and slowly introduced toward the tip/supra-tip, half distance and deep to the medial crurae of the alar cartilages, gently sliding medially through the nasal septum. The injector should see the tip of the cannula discreetly deform the skin of the tip/supra-tip region (**Fig. 8**).

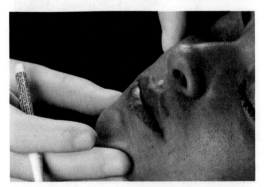

Fig. 3. The white dot marks the philtral entry point of the cannula and is placed approximately 5 mm distal to the columellar-labial junction.

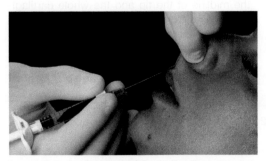

Fig. 5. The nondominant hand is pulling the columella away from the ANS.

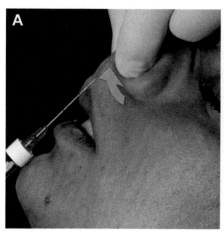
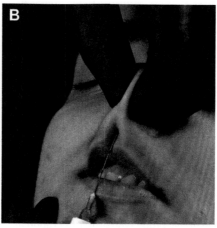

Fig. 6. The nondominant hand is performing a rotational, "crowbar," movement (*green arrow*) of the columella. Lateral (*A*) and oblique (*B*) views.

Once the cannula is positioned at the desired aesthetic location, the alar cartilages should be pressed against each other, halfway down the alares, preventing any reflux of the filler through the cannula pathway. Small boli of 0.05 to 0.1 mL are injected whereby needed (Video 5). The cannula is withdrawn and only then the fingertips squeezing the cartilages are removed.

A distinct ligament between the footplate of the medial crus and the caudal septum does not exist.[22] That allows the cannula to access and move freely through the septum. Following this particular trajectory, the blunt cannula delicately pierces the intercrural ligament at a safer 90-degree angle and reaches the deep fatty layer (**Fig. 9**), as it also avoids the other important ligaments of the tip.

After Steps 1 to 3 are completed, the philtrum skin is pulled in the cephalic direction, against the ANS. This maneuver aims to extract any filler that may have been inadvertently infiltrated into the subcutaneous plane (Video 6).

Step 4 – the Radix and the Nasofrontal Angle

Using the lateral entry point on the nasal dorsum, the cannula is inserted toward the midline, "scraping" the bone, deep to the muscle (**Fig. 10**). The supraperiosteal layer can be tested by trying to lift the cannula, which must be rigidly stationed submuscularly. The bending of the cannula should resemble that of a fishing rod (**Fig. 11**). With the cannula orifice positioned in the midline, a bolus of 0.05 to 0.2 mL is slowly injected (Video 7). Even when aiming to correct a crooked nose, it is possible to still inject at the (safer) midline and then delicately mold the filler to the lateral dorsum, with satisfactory results (**Fig. 12**). Other entry points should be created if more regions of the bony dorsum need treatment. The cannula or needle

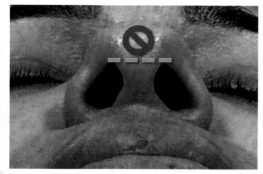

Fig. 7. Illustration of the highest point whereby nostrils connect (*green line*). The red warning sign is indicating the infra-tip region which should not be injected.

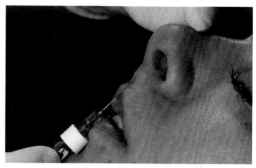

Fig. 8. The tip- and supra-tip region can be accessed through the philtral entry point. The cannula tip can be seen discreetly as a small hump on the nasal dorsum.

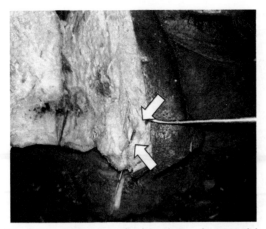

Fig. 9. The anatomic probe (visualizing the cannula), pierces the dorsal portion of the intercrural ligament in a preferred 90-degree angle to reach the deep fatty layer (*white arrows*).

should not move in parallel with the direction of the blood vessel.[23]

Postprocedure care and recommendations

Following a first glance at the nose using a mirror and some remarks and highlights by the physician, a dressing, using 1 cm diameter micropore tape, is placed (**Fig. 13**) for 24 hours, then removed, preferably back in the clinic. The final orientations are given, predominantly about edema (5–10 days) and pain (absent or mild, but present if the nose is hit, especially at the nasolabial angle). No corticosteroids, antibiotics, or painkillers are routinely used, but they can be prescribed in individual cases.

RESULTS
Study Sample and Treatment History

The investigated study sample consisted of a total of 338 patients with a mean age of 38.26 ± 12.49 years [Range: 18–80 years] and a

total number of 511 liquid rhinoplasty procedures, 65 times in male patients and 446 times in females. Step 1, on the anterior nasal spine, was performed in 476 (93.15%) of the treatments; Step 2, columella, 475 (92.95%); Step 3, tip/supra-tip, in 429 (83.95%); and Step 4, nasofrontal angle, in 445 (87.08%) of the procedures. In 173 procedures (33%,84%), the patient had previously undergone liquid rhinoplasty one or more times. In 105 (20.54%) of those times with a collagen-stimulating filler (polymethylmetacrilate or calcium hydroxylapatite), and in 68 (13.30%) with hyaluronic acid (HA). Additionally, in 48 of those treatments (9.39%) the patient had previously been submitted to surgical rhinoplasty. Patient demographics and treatment history are summarized in **Table 1**.

Filler Category and Injected Volume

A total of 266 (52.05%) of the treatments used polymethymetacrilate (PMMA, 30%) + carboxymethylcellulose gels; 230 (45.00%) used distinct HA fillers; 11 (2.15%) treatments were conducted with calcium hydroxyapatite (CH) + carboxymethylcellulose gels; and 1 (0.19%) treatment administered a polycaprolactone + carboxymethylcellulose gel. The average filler amount used was 0.76 ± 0.29 mL. Considered separately, patients who used PMMA were injected with an average of 0.81 ± 0.31 mL, while patients with AH and CH received a lower amount of product, on average: 0.77 ± 0.3 mL and 0.7 ± 0.24 mL, respectively.

Adverse Events

Adverse events reported by patients were documented. Mild phlogistic signs lasting up to 5 days and ecchymosis were not included, as they may be considered usual constituents of the patient's recovery.[24] Using this criterion, 14

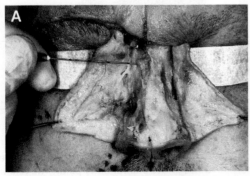
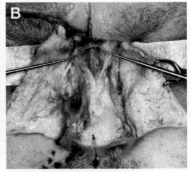

Fig. 10. Anatomic fresh frozen cadaver-dissection demonstrating: (*A*) the cannula insertion under the muscle using the lateral entry point to the bony dorsum; and (*B*) placement of injected filler material (*green*).

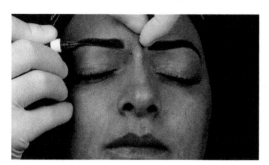

Fig. 11. The cannula placement under the muscle can be tested by applying tension, so that its bending resembles that of a fishing rod.

(2.73%) of the patients experienced adverse effects. Among those, all but one had been treated with PMMA. Three patients developed a visible nodule in the dorsum, while one presented hard, palpable nodules in multiple sites of the nose, and another patient formed a small nodule in the septum, near the anterior nasal spine. All of this occurred approximately 3 to 6 months after the liquid rhinoplasty with PMMA. Three other subjects presented local edema that persisted for a longer period than expected; all had a spontaneous resolution in a few days. One of the patients presented telangiectasias in the nasal tip, perceived 2 months after her third PMMA injection, and was treated with intense pulsed light. Within 24 hours after the procedure, a small amount of

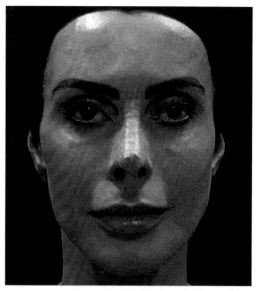

Fig. 13. Postinterventional placement of 1 cm diameter micropore tape on the patient's nose to immobilize and protect the soft-tissue filler and the treated tissues.

the filler extruded through the puncture orifice in the philtrum in one of the patients, while in 2 other cases, also using PMMA, a hardened papule formed at the puncture point in the philtrum after 4 weeks. An additional patient reported an asymmetry in the nasal dorsum observed after the procedure and one last patient, treated with HA, developed a horizontal wrinkle above the upper lip and needed to be injected with hyaluronidase. None of the patients with adverse effects were in the group that had undergone surgical rhinoplasty before the liquid rhinoplasty. Patient demographics and reported adverse events are summarized in **Tables 2** and **3**.

DISCUSSION

Nonsurgical or liquid rhinoplasty, as much as a primary intervention for changing nasal appearance, may also be used to ameliorate slight imperfections or irregularities after surgical rhinoplasty. A systematic review organized by Williams and colleagues[25] concluded that the most common filler used was HA, and a technique that usually involves the application or injection of a local anesthetic followed by the injection of small amounts of product (droplets or linear retrograde threading) using blunt cannulas or needles to deposit the filler, most frequently in the supraperiosteal or supraperichondrial layers. The deep columellar approach technique warrants a safer and reproducible filler injection under the fibromuscular

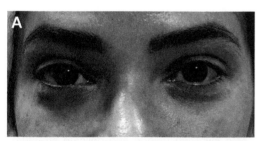

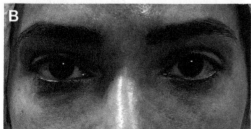

Fig. 12. Treatment results of a female patient with a crooked nose. Before (*A*) and after (*B*) the soft-tissue filler material was placed in the "safer" midline and afterward molded in a more lateral position to correct the lateral deviation of the patient's nose.

Table 2
Patient demographics summary

	Number	Percentage
Gender		
Male	65	12.72%
Female	446	87.28%
Number of Treatments		
One	338	66.14%
Two	134	26.22%
Three	33	6.45%
Four	6	1.17%
Steps Treated		
Step 1	476	93.15%
Step 2	475	92.95%
Step 3	429	83.95%
Step 4	445	87.08%
All Steps (in a single procedure)	462	90.41%
Previous Treatments		
Surgical Rhinoplasty	48	9.39%
AH Liquid Rhinoplasty	68	13.30%
PMMA/CH Liquid Rhinoplasty	105	20.54%
Filler		
Polymethymetacrilate	266	52.05%
Hyaluronic Acid	230	45.00%
Calcium Hydroxyapatite	11	2.15%
Polycaprolactone	1	0.19%

Abbreviations: CH, calcium hydroxylapatite; HA, hyaluronic acid; PMMA, polymethymetacrilate.

Table 3
Adverse events summary

Adverse Event	Area	Filler	Cases	Percentage
Visible Nodule	Dorsum	PMMA	3	0.59%
Palpable Nodule	Nasolabial Junction	PMMA	1	0.20%
Multiple Palpable Nodule	Multiple	PMMA	1	0.20%
Moderate Edema	Nasolabial Junction	PMMA	3	0.59%
Filler Extrusion	Philtrum	PMMA	1	0.20%
Puncture Point Papule	Philtrum	PMMA	2	0.39%
Telangectasias	Tip	PMMA	1	0.20%
Asymmetry	Dorsum	PMMA	1	0.20%
Horizontal Wrinkle	Upper Lip	HA	1	0.20%
Total			14	2.74%

Abbreviations: HA, hyaluronic acid; PMMA, polymethymetacrilate.

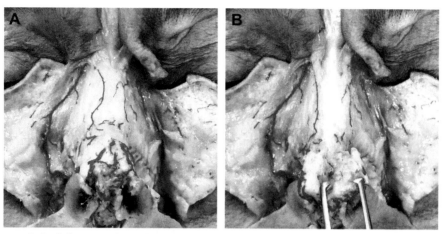

Fig. 14. Anatomic fresh frozen cadaver-dissection showing the fatty layers of the nasal tip: (*A*) the subcutaneous layer (Layer 2) populated by large vessels; and (*B*) the injected gel (light blue) placed exclusively in the deep layer of loose suprapericondrial areolar tissue (Layer 4), using the deep columellar approach.

layer (Video 8), in the less vascularized suprapericondrial layer (**Fig. 14**). Accessing the nose through an infra-tip entry point with a cannula directed cranially, although ergonomically easier, might risk the precise identification of the submuscular layer,[26] [29]threaten the delicate ligaments of the nasal tip and allow the filler to reflow effortlessly to the infra-tip and rectify the columellar-lobular angle or insinuate into the skin at the incision point, preventing cicatrization. This longitudinal course of the cannula, parallel to the lateral dorsal arteries, may also be implicated in cases of visual loss after nasal soft tissue filler injections using cannulas.[29] Overall, the patient satisfaction rate with NSR seems to be over 90%, with a slight decline in satisfaction after 6 months, although it was still over 90%, regardless of the injection technique used.[24,25,27,28] Patients will likely require

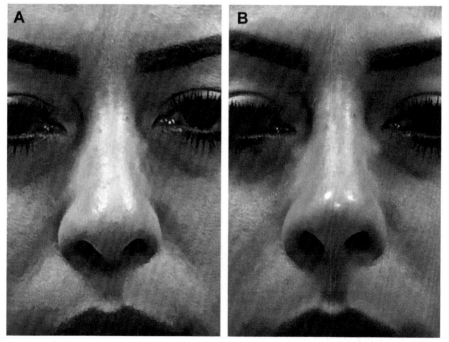

Fig. 15. Placement of soft-tissue filler material in the deep fatty layer can also be effective in nose tip definition as seen by the treatment results of a female patient, before (*A*) and immediately after treatment (*B*).

repeated injections within 12 months to maintain results, but it is not rare to find the shape of the nose has not completely returned to its pretreatment form beyond this period.[6] Once our focus was on the vascular occlusion safety of a particular injection technique, our data did not consider treatment longevity or patient satisfaction. When proposing to treat the supraperiosteal and supraperichondrial layers, one must not forget that, although the deep injections are safer, it is possible that the superficial deposition of the filler could result in a more effective augmentation,[23] especially for tip definition. Nevertheless, we were able to achieve very satisfactory results using the deep columellar approach, even for tip definition (**Fig. 15**).

SUMMARY

Typically, the arteries of the nose course in the superficial fatty layer (Layer 2). Severe complications such as an accidental injection into arteries with retrograde occlusion can effectively be prevented by injecting in the deep fatty layer (Layer 4). The "Deep Columellar Approach" injection algorithm presented in this article offers a safe, effective, reproducible, and reliable method for nose augmentation in liquid rhinoplasty with soft-tissue fillers. The low rate of 2.74% and the low severity of reported adverse events can be drawn back to the precise and verifiable soft-tissue filler placement in the deep fatty layers (supraperiosteal and supraperichondrial), using blunt cannulas.

CLINICS CARE POINTS

- The keys to safety in NSR can be referred to as maintaining the midline of the nose during cannula advancement, the use of blunt cannulas, and precise, low pressure, low volume, filler injection into the deep layers (supraperiosteal or supraperichondrial).

- The deep columellar approach technique warrants a safer and reproducible filler injection under the fibromuscular layer, in the less vascularized supraperichondrial layer.

- A caudal cannula insertion point is used to treat the midline of the tip and the whole cartilaginous nasal dorsum.

- A lateral cannula entry point is used to correct the nasofrontal angle when needed.

SUPPLEMENTARY DATA

Supplementary data related to this article can be found online at https://doi.org/10.1016/j.fsc.2022.01.005.

REFERENCES

1. Springer IN, Zernial O, Nölke F, et al. Gender and nasal shape: Measures for rhinoplasty. Plast Reconstr Surg 2008;121(2):629–37.
2. Chait LA, Widgerow AD. In search of the ideal nose. Plast Reconstr Surg 2000;105(7):2561–7.
3. Oliphant TJ, Langtry JAA. Nasal anatomy for the dermatological surgeon. Br J Dermatol 2014;171(SUPPL. 2):2–6.
4. Furtado IR. Nasal morphology - harmony and proportion applied to rhinoplasty. Rev Bras Cir Plást 2016;31(4):599–608.
5. Perkins SW, Shadfar S. Complications in reductive profileplasty. Facial Plast Surg 2019;35(05):476–85.
6. Harb A, Brewster CT. The nonsurgical rhinoplasty: a retrospective review of 5000 treatments. Plast Reconstr Surg 2020;145(3):661–7.
7. Johnson O, Kontis T. Nonsurgical Rhinoplasty. Facial Plast Surg 2016;32(05):500–6.
8. Rohrich RJ, Agrawal N, Avashia Y, et al. Safety in the use of fillers in nasal augmentation - the liquid rhinoplasty. Plast Reconstr Surg - Glob Open 2020;8(8):e2820.
9. Jasin ME. Nonsurgical rhinoplasty using dermal fillers. Facial Plast Surg Clin North Am 2013;21(2):241–52.
10. Humphrey CD, Arkins JP, Dayan SH. Soft tissue fillers in the nose. Aesthet Surg J 2009;29(6):477–84.
11. Rzany B, DeLorenzi C. Understanding, avoiding, and managing severe filler complications. Plast Reconstr Surg 2015;136(5):196S–203S.
12. Bertossi D, Lanaro L, Dell'Acqua I, et al. Injectable profiloplasty: Forehead, nose, lips, and chin filler treatment. J Cosmet Dermatol 2019;18(4):976–84.
13. Colombo G, Caregnato P, Stifanese R, et al. A vast intranasal filler-induced granulomatous reaction: A case report. Aesthet Plast Surg 2010;34(5):660–3.
14. Chen Q, Liu Y, Fan D. Serious vascular complications after nonsurgical rhinoplasty. Plast Reconstr Surg - Glob Open 2016;4(4):e683.
15. Lee J il, Kang SJ, Sun H. Skin necrosis with oculomotor nerve palsy due to a hyaluronic acid filler injection. Arch Plast Surg 2017;44(4):340–3.
16. Beleznay K, Carruthers JDA, Humphrey S, et al. Update on avoiding and treating blindness from fillers: a recent review of the world literature. Aesthet Surg J 2019;39(6):662–74.

17. Kim EG, Eom TK, Kang SJ. Severe visual loss and cerebral infarction after injection of hyaluronic acid gel. J Craniofac Surg 2014;25(2):684–6.

18. Tasman A-J. Rhinoplasty - indications and techniques. GMS Curr Top Otorhinolaryngol Head Neck Surg 2007;6:Doc09.

19. Tasman A-J. Rhinoplasty photography: lighting from above improves visualization of deviations and irregularities. Facial Plast Surg Aesthet Med 2020;X(X):1–6.

20. Saban Y, Amodeo CA, Hammou JC, et al. An anatomical study of the nasal superficial musculoaponeurotic system. Arch Facial Plast Surg 2008;10(2):109–15.

21. Goh S, Karamchandani D, Anari S. Relationship of the posterior septal angle to the anterior nasal spine in the Caucasian nasal septum. J Laryngol Otol 2019;133(03):224–6.

22. Daniel RK, Palhazi P. The nasal ligaments and tip support in rhinoplasty: an anatomical study. Aesthet Surg J 2018;38(4):357–68.

23. Jung GS, Chu SG, Lee JW, et al. A safer non-surgical filler augmentation rhinoplasty based on the anatomy of the nose. Aesthet Plast Surg 2019;43(2):447–52.

24. Kumar V, Jain A, Atre S, et al. Non-surgical rhinoplasty using hyaluronic acid dermal fillers: A systematic review. J Cosmet Dermatol 2021;20(8):2414–24.

25. Williams LC, Kidwai SM, Mehta K, et al. Nonsurgical rhinoplasty: a systematic review of technique, outcomes, and complications. Plast Reconstr Surg 2020;146(1):41–51.

26. Rosengaus F, Nikolis A. Cannula versus needle in medical rhinoplasty: the nose knows. J Cosmet Dermatol 2020;19(12):3222–8.

27. Rauso R, Colella G, Zerbinati N, et al. Safety and early satisfaction assessment of patients seeking nonsurgical rhinoplasty with filler. J Cutan Aesthet Surg 2017;10(4):207.

28. Radulesco T, de Bonnecaze G, Penicaud M, et al. Patient satisfaction after non-surgical rhinoplasty using hyaluronic acid: a literature review. Aesthet Plast Surg 2021;45(6):2896–901.

29. Alfertshofer Michael G, Konstantin Frank, Ehrl Denis, et al. The Layered Anatomy of the Nose: An Ultrasound-Based Investigation. Aesthetic Surgery Journal 2021;42(4):349–57. https://doi.org/10.1093/asj/sjab310.

Deep Plane Anatomy for the Facelift Surgeon
A Comprehensive Three-Dimensional Journey

Christopher C. Surek, DO, FACS[a],*, Amanda Moorefield, BS[b]

KEYWORDS

• Face • Facelift • SMAS • Retaining Ligament • Facial Nerve • Deep Plane Facelift

KEY POINTS

• The face is divided in 5 key anatomical layers, deep plane facelift surgery occurs in Layer 4. The sub-SMAS layer.
• The facial nerve branches have an intimate relationship with the retaining ligaments.
• The Great Auricular Nerve can be triangulated by marking a vertical line through the ear lobule paired with an oblique line 30 degrees posterior to it. This demarcates the region of the nerves pathway.

Abbreviations	
Facelift	deep Plane Anatomy

INTRODUCTION

The deep plane facelift surgeon must develop a sense of spatial awareness and navigation within the intricate anatomy of the face and neck, and this requires an understanding of 3-dimensional layering and depth. Simplistically, one can separate the face into 5 layers based on depth and into lateral and anterior components based on function. A vertical line drawn from the lateral orbital rim through the mandible demarcates the anterior (mobile) component from the lateral (immobile) component of the face; this correlates with the line of underlying retaining ligaments that connect the overlying skin to the bone and/or deep fascial layers.[1–11] The lateral face is relatively immobile because the structures in this region are designed for mastication requiring much less emphasis on precise movement, whereas the anterior face requires significant mobility to facilitate communication and expression.[1,3–7,9,11–14]

Layers 1 through 3 of the mid and lower face consist of the skin (epidermis and dermis), the subcutaneous layer (subcutaneous fat and the retinacular cutis), and the superficial musculoaponeurotic system (SMAS), which together work as a composite flap to move over the deep fascia of layer 5.[1,7] Layer 3 is continuous over the entire face with the main focus of facelift surgery, the SMAS, covering the portion of the mid and lower face.[1,5–7,9,10,15–19] These layers are considered safe for dissection because the complexity and potential danger arises in sub-SMAS territory. Layer 4 of the anterior face contains the retaining ligaments, deep fat compartments, and facial soft tissue spaces that help orchestrate movement, whereas layer 4 of the lateral face serves primarily as a region of fusion.[1–5] Layer 5 consists of either periosteum positioned over bony

a Surek Plastic Surgery, Kansas City University, University of Kansas Medical Center; b Kansas City University
* Corresponding author. 7901 W. 135th StreetOverland Park, KS 66223.
E-mail address: Csurek@gmail.com

Facial Plast Surg Clin N Am 30 (2022) 205–214
https://doi.org/10.1016/j.fsc.2022.01.015
1064-7406/22/
© 2022 Elsevier Inc. All rights reserved.

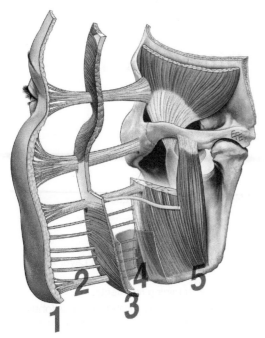

Fig. 1. Illustrative diagram of the 5-layer arrangement of the face. Layer 1 contains the epidermis and dermis. Layer 2 (subcutaneous layer) contains the superficial fat compartments and retinacular cutis. Layer 3 contains the SMAS, galea, orbicularis fascia, superficial temporal fascia, and platysma. Layer 4 contains facial nerve branches, retaining ligaments, deep fat compartments, and potential spaces. Layer 5 contains periosteum over bony locations or deep fascia covering muscles that overlie the bone.

locations or deep fascia when covering muscles that overlie the bone (**Figs. 1–3**).

A comprehensive understanding of how aging impacts facial anatomy is crucial for proper patient assessment and preoperative planning, including but not limited to, changes to skin quality and composition, the loss of adiposity, volumetric deflation, tissue descent, and changes to the facial skeleton.[20] Patient assessment should include an analysis of the patient's skin quality, including Fitzpatrick skin type, their facial shape, and the presence or absence of asymmetries.[7,20] Evaluation of the midcheek includes the degree of segmentation of the malar, nasolabial, and lid cheek segments, noting evidence of malar pad descent with malar volume depletion and fullness of the submalar region.[9–15,21] Other findings to look for are skin redundancy, nasolabial fold prominence, marionette lines, and evident jowling. The contour of the jawline and neck should also be evaluated making note of platysma laxity, the presence of vertical banding, or submental and submandibular fat prominence.

Although understanding the nuances of the aging face is vital, the patient assessment should first and foremost be guided by identifying the patient's main concerns and addressing features they find most bothersome. It is crucial that the facelift surgeon practices a patient-centered approach in which surgical plans are individualized based on his or her expertise and the patient's expectations.[20] Patient planning includes more than facial analysis, but it also requires comprehensive evaluation of the patient's medical history, medication list, anesthesia history, as well as a psychosocial evaluation.[20]

METHODS

This is a single-surgeon narrative review based on the experience of the senior author and does not include a full literature review or data analysis.

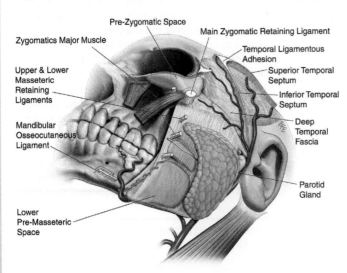

Fig. 2. Illustration of layers 4 and 5 of the face. These layers contain deep facial fascia, retaining ligaments, septa, adhesions, and potential spaces.

Pre-Zygomatic Space
Zygomatics Major Muscle
Upper & Lower Masseteric Retaining Ligaments
Mandibular Osseocutaneous Ligament
Lower Pre-Masseteric Space
Main Zygomatic Retaining Ligament
Temporal Ligamentous Adhesion
Superior Temporal Septum
Inferior Temporal Septum
Deep Temporal Fascia
Parotid Gland

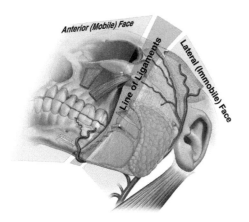

Fig. 3. Illustration of the anterior and lateral components of the face divided by the line of retaining ligaments.

The aim of this review is to provide pearls for patient assessment of the facelift candidate, for preoperative planning, and to discuss the pertinent anatomy of sub-SMAS facelift technique for safe and effective surgical execution.

Facial Depth: Why the Facial Layers Matter for the Surgeon

The sub-SMAS layers (4 and 5) are critical areas for the surgeon to be familiar with in extended SMAS dissection, because the facial nerve branches pass from deep to superficial within layer 4.[1,3,7,9,16] All the facial nerve branches exit the parotid gland at the deep fascial level of the lateral face known as the parotid-masseteric fascia and become more superficial in the anterior face. The parotid-masseteric fascia is found below the zygomatic arch where it also covers the parotid gland with the deep temporal fascia extending cranially beyond the zygomatic arch. The deep fascial layer located caudally over the submandibular space and suprahyoid muscles is referred to as the deep cervical fascia.[1,3–10,17–19] The superficial muscles of the face such as the frontalis, orbicularis oculi, and the platysma muscles have minimal direct attachment to the underlying skeleton.[1,13] Owing to this more superficial location, stabilization is primarily ensured by vertical retaining ligaments such as the superior temporal septum, the lateral orbital thickening, and the lower masseteric ligament.[1,8,11,13]

The platysma-auricular fascia (PAF) lies in layer 4 of the lateral face representing the largest area of ligamentous attachment serving as a good option for surgical fixation.[1,3–6,8,11] The PAF arises from the parotid fascia extending anterior to the ear and is an important landmark because the tail of the parotid gland can be found more superficially in this region. The fascial attachment anterior to the tragus has been termed Lore fascia.[1,22,23] The platysma-auricular ligament (PAL) extends from the posterior border of the platysma to the inferior auricular region connecting the platysma to the SMAS layer superiorly and to the sternocleidomastoid fascia caudally around the earlobe.[1–3,7,24] Both fascial structures can be used for platysma suspension sutures during platysmaplasty.[23] However, caution must be taken in this region because the great auricular nerve is close to the posterior border of the platysma with some of the cutaneous branches coursing through the PAL.[1–3,7,24]

Layer 4 is the plane of dissection for extended SMAS facelift technique. Key benefits of this plane include the avascular nature of the areola tissue, which allows the surgeon to minimize blood loss; reduction of postoperative bruising and swelling; as well as the ease of separation during dissection from the underlying periosteum.[1] Although there are many advantages to dissecting in this plane, it is not without risk, because the facial nerve branches innervate the mimetic muscles of the face after coursing from deep to superficial within layer 4.[1,7,15,16,19,25,26]

The Significance of Superficial Musculoaponeurotic System

SMAS belongs to layer 3 in the region of the mid and lower face serving as the midface cranial extension of the platysma and caudal extension of the superficial temporal fascia.[1,5–7,9,10,15–18] The superficial temporal fascia is also known as the temporoparietal fascia and begins at the level of the zygomatic arch blending with the frontalis muscles, the galea aponeurotica, as well as the orbicularis oculi.[1,4–7,10] When undermining the skin flap during facelifting, it is paramount that the surgeon frequently checks the plane of dissection. Dissection superficial to SMAS is considered a safe zone; however, extended SMAS dissection with ligamentous release allows the facelift surgeon to have increased viability for long-term control with an enhanced aesthetic result.[1,7] As the surgeon delves into the sub-SMAS plane it is crucial that the surgeon is confident with the facial nerve pathways and their relationship to the layered anatomy.

The facial retaining ligaments are cylindrical fibrous structures that connect the superficial layers of the face and the SMAS with the deeper tissues. Mendelson[16] described the retaining ligament system as a "tree-like" distribution with each ligament rooted into the periosteum like the trunk of tree with branching occurring as one approaches the SMAS and travels superficially toward the skin.[1] (**Fig. 4**). The region of "branching" in the subcutaneous fat

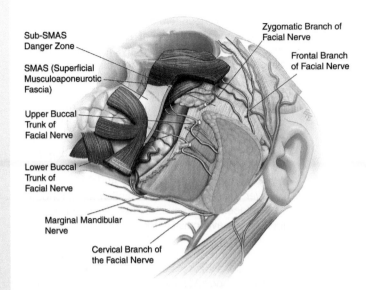

Sub-SMAS Danger Zone

SMAS (Superficial Musculoaponeurotic Fascia)

Upper Buccal Trunk of Facial Nerve

Lower Buccal Trunk of Facial Nerve

Marginal Mandibular Nerve

Cervical Branch of the Facial Nerve

Zygomatic Branch of Facial Nerve

Frontal Branch of Facial Nerve

Fig. 4. Illustration of layer 3 of the face composed of the SMAS. Note the course of all 5 facial nerve branches beginning deep in layer 4 and then traversing more superficially with vertical path of the retaining ligaments.

is known as the retinacular cutis[8,11] and contributes to the formation of septa,[8,11,17] which in turn divides the subcutaneous fat of the face into compartments.[8,11]

The Retaining Ligaments

The retaining ligaments of the face are discussed in detail throughout the literature but with discontinuity in authors' preferred classification system and nomenclature. In effort to minimize confusion, when describing the retaining ligaments, we focus on the distinction between true versus false retaining ligaments. The mandibular and zygomatic ligaments are true retaining ligaments, distinguished as osteocutaneous ligaments, which connect the skin through all fascial layers to the underlying bone. The masseteric ligaments are false retaining ligaments, also termed fasciocutaneous ligaments, which connect the skin to the deeper fascial layers but lack any attachment to bone.[6,18]

True retaining ligaments

The mandibular ligament or mandibular osteocutaneous ligament (MOCL) holds the superficial layers of the face to the anterior mandible just above the boundary between the SMAS and platysma anteriorly.[1–4,7,10–13,22] The MOCL demarcates a transition from the labiomandibular fold superiorly to the jowl.[1] The mandibular ligament maintains a lot of its strength with aging, and thus can become more apparent as the surrounding tissues increase in laxity creating an area of shackling. The zygomatic ligament originates at the inferior border of the zygomatic arch and extends along the arch and body of the zygoma with the main zygomatic

ligament located just lateral to the zygomaticus major muscle. The region of the zygomatic ligaments that travel through the malar fat pad is known as McGregor patch.[1–4,7,10–13,22] Transverse facial artery perforators can exist in this patch leading to occasional bleeding following ligament release. Both the mandibular and zygomatic ligaments require a sharp release for dissection. Both ligamentous releases can contribute significantly to final tissue draping and overall improved esthetic outcome.[1,7,8,11]

False retaining ligaments

The masseteric ligaments are a series of ligaments overlying the masseter muscle that hold the SMAS to the masseteric fascia.[1,7] The masseteric ligaments separate the lateral cheek compartment and the premasseter space over the lower masseter.[27] The upper masseteric ligament is often released in sub-SMAS dissection while leaving the lower masseteric ligament unreleased due to its relationship to the buccal fat pad.[7,16,18,27–31] The weakening of the masseteric ligaments is implicated as the anatomic explanation for the formation of jowls with aging.[1–5,7,9,10,25] The platysma mandibular ligament originates at the anterior border of the masseter muscle along the mandibular border, lying 9 mm inferior and lateral to the mandibular ligament, and attaches the platysma-SMAS layer to the mandible.[7,12,24]

The Potential Spaces for the Facelift Surgeon

Mendelson and Wong[32] defined soft tissue spaces based on the following key characteristics:

- Well-defined membranous boundaries and retaining ligaments
- Nerves and vasculature located between spaces
- Absence of vital structures within or coursing across the spaces.

The absence of vital structures and avascular nature of the spaces provides safe surgical access to various regions of the face for sub-SMAS dissection.[1,7,32–34] These spaces are not only key regions for surgical access but also play a significant role in the aging face. The fascial spaces are close together in youth and slowly expand as we age, which occurs at a greater degree than the laxity observed in the retaining ligaments; this creates areas of irregularity within and between the spaces due to overall laxity of the compartment against areas of fixation.[1–4,7–9,17,24]

Prezygomatic space

The prezygomatic space overlies the body of the zygoma with the superior border formed by the orbicularis retaining ligament (ORL) and inferiorly bound by the medial border of the zygomatic ligaments (also known as zygomaticocutaneous ligaments).[1,2,10,14] The roof of the prezygomatic area is suborbicularis oculi fat (SOOF), and the floor is formed by preperiosteal fat and bone.[1] Blunt dissection into this space can be used to mobilize the midface during facelift surgery.

Lower premasseteric space

The lower premasseteric space is rhomboid and overlies the lower half of the masseter immediately anterior to the parotid. The roof of the space is formed by the platysma muscle.[1,33,34] The posterior border is defined by the posterior auricular ligament, and the anterior border is reinforced by the masseteric ligaments. The effects of aging on the lower premasseter space are quite notable because this space is associated with the development of jowls and deep labiomandibular folds. Significant laxity can be observed with aging in the masseteric ligaments of the anterior masseter. Even more dramatic effect is observed at the inferior boundary of the lower premasseteric space where no ligament is present.[1,3–7,32–35] Weakening of the roof of the space and enlargement of the space in general can cause sinking of the roof of the premasseteric space creating a prominent jowl effect. In addition, distention of the weaker masseteric ligaments and wit and buccal fat prolapse within the buccal space contributes to prominent labiomandibular folds.[7,9,13,32–34,36]

The 3-dimensional Journey of the Facial Nerve

Spatial recognition is crucial for the facelift surgeon because the facial nerve courses through the facial layers at varying depths. The retaining ligaments are key markers for identifying transition points as the facial nerve branches traverse from deep to superficial.[2,7,12,22,27] These areas of facial nerve traversing are at high risk of injury.[1] The frontal and mandibular branches are the most significant in terms of surgical risks because they have limited have limiinterconnections with the other facial nerve branches.[7] The most injured branch is the buccal branch of the facial nerve, although patients are usually asymptomatic due to the extensive network of rami contributing to one's smile.[7,37,38]

Frontal branch

After leaving the superior surface of the parotid gland, the frontal rami (also known as the temporal branch) of the facial nerve can be found using Pitanguy[35] line, which extends from a point 0.5 cm inferior to the tragus to a point 1.5 cm lateral to the supraorbital rim.[1,7,37–40] Another topographic marking is a point 4 cm lateral to the lateral canthus at the level of the helical root. The frontal rami travel along the middle third of the zygomatic arch deep to the orbital rim and transition to the underside of the superficial temporal fascia (layer 3) at least 1.5 to 3 cm above the zygomatic arch.[1,7] This transition occurs before the frontal branch reaches the sentinel vein. There can be 3-5 rami. The rami commonly travel along the inferior temporal septum along with an anterior branch of the superficial temporal artery (**Fig. 5**). Further superiorly, the frontal rami transition superficially at the SMAS level to reach the underside of orbicularis oculi and the frontalis muscles.[7,40,41]

Zygomatic branch

The zygomatic branches of the facial nerve are located caudal to the zygomatic ligaments. The zygomatic branch exits the parotid gland just inferior to the zygoma and inferior to the parotid duct.[7,40,41] The zygomatic nerve travels horizontally on the masseter with the transverse facial artery.[42,43] The lower zygomatic nerve is more superficial than the upper zygomatic nerve with the upper masseteric ligament positioned between the upper and lower zygomatic rami.[7,26]

Before entering the zygomaticus major muscle in the inferolateral corner, the zygomatic nerve gives off a branch to the orbicularis oculi muscle.[6,14,39] The zygomatic branch then transitions to the underside of zygomaticus major to innervate the zygomaticus major and minor muscles from layer 4. The zygomatic branches are located

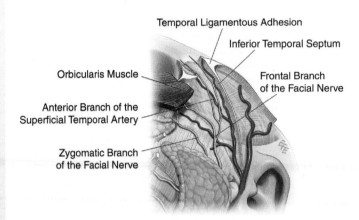

Temporal Ligamentous Adhesion

Inferior Temporal Septum

Orbicularis Muscle

Frontal Branch
of the Facial Nerve

Anterior Branch of the
Superficial Temporal Artery

Zygomatic Branch
of the Facial Nerve

Fig. 5. Illustration of the path of the frontal branch of the facial nerve. The nerve contains 3 to 5 rami, some of which will run along the inferior temporal septum in proximity of an anterior branch of the superficial temporal artery.

caudal to the zygomatic ligaments and anterior to the masseteric ligaments, which is why the region 1 cm below zygomatic major muscle has been termed a sub-SMAS danger zone.[3,6,7,14,27] For this reason, during an extended SMAS facelift dissection the surgeon should proceed with caution when reaching the origin of the zygomaticus major muscle. The fat immediately inferior to the muscle origin contains zygomatic nerve branches (ie, sub-SMAS danger zone). Dissection should be performed superficial to the muscle to facilitate entrance into the prezygomatic space, and thus avoid nerve injury (**Fig. 6**).

Buccal branches

The buccal branches course in the superior and inferior boundaries of the lower premasseteric space so the surgeon must be able to distinguish the lower premasseteric space from the upper premasseteric space intraoperatively to avoid damaging the nerves. The buccal branches are located caudal to the zygomatic ligaments and anterior to the masseteric ligaments.[3,6,7,14,27] The

upper buccal trunk exits the parotid superficial to the parotid duct and then dives deep to the masseter fascia to continue anteriorly in the deep plane until the edge of the masseter is reached.[6] The upper buccal branch exits the floor of the masseteric fascia traveling vertically with the upper masseteric ligament.[1,6,7,34] The lower buccal trunk leaves the parotid at the level of the earlobe and travels underneath the masseter fascia coursing the floor of the lower premasseteric space. Like the upper buccal branch, the lower buccal branch transitions from deep to the underside of SMAS within the lower masseteric ligament.[1,6,7,34] The upper and lower buccal trunks connect via a communicating branch.

Marginal mandibular branch

Early in its course the marginal mandibular nerve (MMN) leaves the parotid gland at the PAF as it travels along the angle of the mandible. The nerve remains within the PAF as it courses along the inferior boundary of the lower premasseteric space.[1,12] The MMN exits the parotid-masseteric

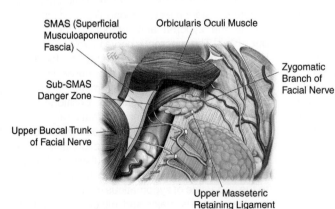

SMAS (Superficial
Musculoaponeurotic
Fascia)

Orbicularis Oculi Muscle

Sub-SMAS
Danger Zone

Zygomatic
Branch of
Facial Nerve

Upper Buccal Trunk
of Facial Nerve

Upper Masseteric
Retaining Ligament

Fig. 6. Illustration of the path of the zygomatic branch of the facial nerve. As the nerve reaches the origin of the zygomaticus major muscle it travels into adipose tissue deep to the muscle; this region is termed the sub-SMAS danger zone because surgical dissection in this plane is at risk for nerve injury. If a surgeon desires to dissect into the prezygomatic space it is recommended to proceed superficial to the zygomaticus major muscle to avoid the sub-SMAS danger zone.

fascia to become sub-SMAS as it crosses the facial vessels. The MMN passes the vessels at one-fourth of the length from the gonial angle to the midline point of the anterior chin.[7,12] The nerve remains in the sub-SMAS plane, deep to the platysma as it continues toward the depressors of the lower lip.[7,12] The MMN passes superficial to the submandibular fascia and the facial vessels but remains deep to the platysma.

The most vulnerable region of the mandibular branch is where it crosses the facial vessels near the anterior mandible. The MMN remains deep to the platysma/SMAS until it reaches the depressor anguli oris muscle[1,4,5,7,12,26,33,35–38,42–45] (**Fig. 7**). Huettner and colleagues[46] recorded that based on their study, the MMN on average had 2 branches. The terminal branch of the MMN always passed superior to the mandibular ligament. In addition, distal to the facial vessels, most of the MMN branches were superior to the mandibular border (81%).[46] After the nerves reach layer 3, the zygomatic, upper and lower buccal trunks, and mandibular branch meet before continuing their course to innervate their respective facial muscles.[1]

Cervical branch

The cervical branch exits the parotid gland and travels inferiorly to supply the platysma. The nerve travels deep to the platysma within at least 1.5 cm of the gonial angle, after which it gives off multiple branches to supply to the platysma in the suprahyoid region.[1,7,47–49]

The Great Auricular Nerve

The great auricular nerve is the most common symptomatic nerve injury during facelift surgery.[50]

The great auricular nerve travels approximately 6.5 cm inferior to the external acoustic meatus, which is often referred as McKinney point.[3,4,51] When dissecting in this region the surgeon must remain superficial to the muscular fascia because the nerves are positioned deep to this point.[3,4,7,12,36,39,51–53] A topographic marking consisting of a vertical line through the ear lobule, perpendicular to Frankfurt horizontal line, paired with an oblique line 30° posterior demarcates the region of the great auricular nerve[7,50] (**Fig. 8**).

The Deep Neck

The neck consists of distinct fat layers. The superficial or supraplatysmal compartment, between the skin and platysma, is the most associated with adipose accumulation.[7,54] The intermediate or subplatysmal fat compartment, between the platysma and anterior digastric muscles, contains less fat and is mostly dense and fibrotic.[7,54,55] The subplatysmal fat is traingular in shape and often resected in deep necklift surgery to improve contour and shape. Submandibular gland ptosis or digastric muscle belly prominence may occur in some patients, especially after correcting the superficial layers of the face.[1,2,6,7,36,56–60] In select patients, dissection of the intermediate compartment of the neck for resection of the anterior digastric bellies and/or the superficial portion of the submandibular gland may be necessary to improve neck contour.[7,11] However, extreme caution must be taken with deep neck dissection because the intermediate space houses extensive blood vessels and lymph tissue.[7,54]

How Does Aging Impact This Anatomy?

Aging occurs at many levels influencing the anatomy of the face in a variety of ways. The skin undergoes

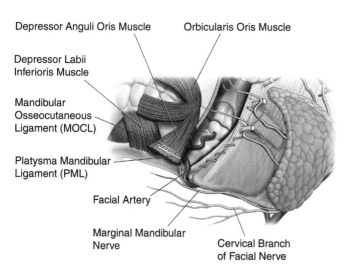

Depressor Anguli Oris Muscle

Orbicularis Oris Muscle

Depressor Labii Inferioris Muscle

Mandibular Osseocutaneous Ligament (MOCL)

Platysma Mandibular Ligament (PML)

Facial Artery

Marginal Mandibular Nerve

Cervical Branch of Facial Nerve

Fig. 7. Illustration of the path of the marginal mandibular branch of the facial nerve (MMN). The MMN leaves parotid masseteric fascia to become sub-SMAS as it crosses the facial vessels superficially and remains deep to the platysma. The MMN innervates the depressor angular oris on the posterior surface and the mentalis muscle on the superficial surface. The MMN travels in proximity to the mandibular ligament. Surgical release of the mandibular ligament and the platysma mandibular ligament (PML) should be performed in the subcutaneous place to avoid inadvertent injury to the MMN.

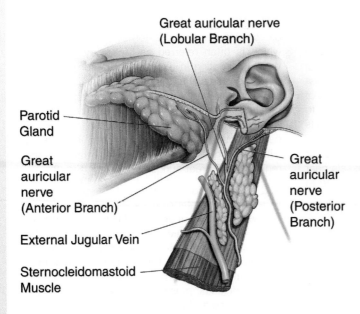

Great auricular nerve
(Lobular Branch)

Parotid
Gland

Great
auricular
nerve
(Anterior Branch)

External Jugular Vein

Sternocleidomastoid
Muscle

Great
auricular
nerve
(Posterior
Branch)

Fig. 8. Illustration of the path of the great auricular nerve (GAN). The GAN travels within the sternocleidomastoid fascia and divides into 3 distinct branches (anterior, lobular, and posterior). A topographic marking using a vertical line through the lobule perpendicular to Frankfurt horizontal line and then an oblique line 30° posterior delineate the area of GAN location. Surgical dissection in this area should be performed carefully above the SCM fascia to avoid inadvertent GAN injury.

many changes with aging such as thinning of the dermal and epidermal layers, loss of elasticity, decreased collagen, pigmentation, dyschromia, decreased adipose tissue, and volumetric deflation.[1] There are various factors that contribute to these skin changes, ranging from sun exposure, smoking, major weight fluctuations, Fitzpatrick skin classification, to the normal aging process.

The facial skeleton is prone to bone resorption with aging primarily involving the orbital rim, the midface such as the maxilla, and the prejowl region of the mandible.[1] Retrusion of the mandible causes the retaining ligaments to shift posteriorly resulting in loss of projection with exaggerated concavities.[9,13,15,29] The 3 segments of the midcheek that become prominent with aging are the nasolabial region, the malar region, and the lid-cheek region.[1] The evident segmentation of these regions contributes to the overall aged and tired appearance.

The prominence of the inferior orbital rim, maxilla bone resorption, and soft tissue decline due to aging all contribute to the orbital fat of the infraorbital rim to be visible on the underside of the lid fat bulge.[1] All these factors contribute to what seems to be a lengthened lower lid-cheek junction.[5–9,55,58,59] Other periocular changes include dermatochalasis, eyelid ptosis, protrusion of the periorbital fat, and brow ptosis.[1] The perioral region also experiences changes with aging evident by a decreased fullness in the upper lip and downturning of the oral commissures.[59,60]

It is imperative to approach the aging face with the general appreciation that aging is multifactorial and patient specific.[61] Although we have addressed numerous anatomic changes that occur with aging, there are a few overarching themes that the extended SMAS technique aims to address: volume loss, tissue descent from their original anatomic plane, skin redundancy, fat displacement, and contour irregularities. The degree and signs of aging will vary greatly from patient to patient. For this reason, some patients may benefit from adjunctive procedures in conjunction with their facelift surgery. Both surgical and nonsurgical procedures, when appropriate, should be openly discussed as options for optimizing the final aesthetic outcome. Although not every patient will be a candidate or desire adjunctive treatment, it is crucial that they are supplied with all the options and details to make a fully informed decision. Open communication and transparency are vital for a successful outcome for both the facelift surgeon and patient.

SUMMARY

Facelift surgery, particularly in the sub-SMAS plane, is a delicate journey within soft tissue spaces, between retaining ligaments and around the 3-dimensional pathways of the facial nerve. Spatial awareness of these structures can aid the surgeon as they navigate ligament release, SMAS elevation, and SMAS repositioning. Treatment of the aging anatomy of the face with a comprehensive, patient-centered, and anatomically based approach can yield predictable and reproducible surgical outcomes.

CLINICS CARE POINTS

- Caution should be excercised in deep plane facelift dissection to avoid injury to the facial nerve branches which have an intimate relationship with the retaining ligaments.

- The potential spaces in the sub-SMAS plane can be useful for blunt dissection and mobilization of a SMAS flap during deep plane facelift surgery.

- Be cogizant of the Great Auricular Nerve depth and location when performing postauricular skin flap elevation.

REFERENCES

1. Mendelson B, Wong CH. Anatomy of the aging face. In: Neligan PC, editor. Plastic surgery. Toronto, Canada: Elsevier; 2013. p. 78–92.

2. Muzaffar AR, Mendelson BC, Adams WP Jr. Surgical anatomy of the ligamentous attachments of the lower lid and lateral canthus. Plast Reconstr Surg 2002;110(3):873–911. https://doi.org/10.1097/00006534-200209010-00025.

3. Furnas DW. The retaining ligaments of the cheek. Plast Reconstr Surg 1989;83(1):11–6. https://doi.org/10.1097/00006534-198901000-00003.

4. Furnas D. The superficial musculoaponeurotic plane and the retaining ligaments of the face. In: Psillakis JM, editor. Deep face-lifting techniques. New York: Thieme Medical; 1994.

5. Mitz V, Peyronie M. The superficial musculoaponeurotic system (SMAS) in the parotid and cheek area. Plast Reconstr Surg 1976;58(1):80–8. https://doi.org/10.1097/00006534-197607000-00013.

6. Stuzin JM, Baker TJ, Gordon HL. The relationship of the superficial and deep facial fascias: relevance to rhytidectomy and aging. Plast Reconstr Surg 1992; 89(3):441–51.

7. Hashem AM, Couto RA, Duraes EFR, et al. Facelift Part I: History, Anatomy, and Clinical Assessment. Aesthet Surg J 2020;40(1):1–18. https://doi.org/10.1093/asj/sjy326.

8. Rohrich RJ, Pessa JE. The retaining system of the face: histologic evaluation of the septal boundaries of the subcutaneous fat compartments. Plast Reconstr Surg 2008;121(5):1804–9.

9. Mendelson BC Jacobson SR. Surgical anatomy of the midcheek: facial layers, spaces and the midcheek segments. Clin Plast Surg 2008;35:395–404.

10. Mohammed Alghoul MD, Mark A, Codner MD. Retaining Ligaments of the Face: Review of Anatomy and Clinical Applications. Aesthet Surg J 2013; 33(Issue 6):769–82.

11. Rohrich RJ, Pessa JE. The fat compartments of the face: anatomy and clinical implications for cosmetic surgery. Plast Reconstr Surg 2007;119(7):2219–27.

12. Huettner F, Rueda S, Ozturk CN, et al. The relationship of the marginal mandibular nerve to the mandibular osseocutaneous ligament and lesser ligaments of the lower face. Aesthet Surg J 2015;35(2):111–20.

13. Mendelson BC. Correction of the nasolabial fold: extended SMAS dissection with periosteal fixation. Plast Reconstr Surg 1992;89(5):822–33.

14. Mendelson BC, Muzaffar AR, Adams WP Jr. Surgical anatomy of the mid-cheek and malar mounds. Plast Reconstr Surg 2002;110(3):885–911.

15. Mendelson BC. Advances in the understanding of the surgical anatomy of the face. In: Eisenmann-Klein M, Neuhann-Lorenz C, editors. Innovations in plastic and aesthetic surgery. New York: Springer Verlag; 2007. p. 141–5.

16. Mendelson BC. Extended sub-SMAS dissection and cheek elevation. Clin Plast Surg 1995;22:325–39.

17. Gosain AK, Yousif NJ, Madiedo G, et al. Surgical anatomy of the SMAS: a reinvestigation. Plast Reconstr Surg 1993;92:1254–65.

18. Stuzin JM, Baker TJ, Gordon HL, et al. Extended SMAS dissection as an approach to midface rejuvenation. Clin Plast Surg 1995;22:295–311.

19. Jost G, Levet Y. Parotid fascia and face lifting: a critical evaluation of the SMAS concept. Plast Reconstr Surg 1984;74(1):42–51.

20. Santosa KB, Oliver JD, Thompson G, et al. Perioperative Management of the Facelift Patient. Clin Plast Surg 2019;46(4):625–39. https://doi.org/10.1016/j.cps.2019.06.008.

21. Ghavami A, Pessa JE, Janis J, et al. The orbicularis retaining ligament of the medial orbit: closing the circle. Plast Reconstr Surg 2008;121(3):994–1001.

22. Moss CJ, Mendelson BC, Taylor GI. Surgical anatomy of the ligamentous attachments in the temple and periorbital regions. Plast Reconstr Surg 2000; 105(4):1475–90.

23. O'Brien JX, Rozen WM, Whitaker IS, et al. Lore's fascia and the platysma-auricular ligament are distinct structures. J Plast Reconstr Aesthet Surg 2012;65(9): e241–5. https://doi.org/10.1016/j.bjps.2012.03.007.

24. Feldman JJ. Surgical anatomy of the neck. In: Feldman JJ, editor. Necklift. 1st edition. Stuttgart, Germany: Thieme; 2006. p. 106–13.

25. Mendelson BC. Facelift anatomy, SMAS, retaining ligaments and facial spaces. In: Aston J, Steinbrech DS, Walden JL, editors. Aesthetic plastic surgery. London: Saunders Elsevier; 2009. p. 53–72.

26. Seckel BR. Facial danger zones: Avoiding nerve injury in facial Plastic surgery. St Louis: Quality Medical; 1994.

27. Alghoul M, Bitik O, McBride J, et al. Relationship of the zygomatic facial nerve to the retaining ligaments of the face: the Sub-SMAS danger zone. Plast Reconstr Surg 2013;131(2):245e–52e.

28. Warren RJ, Aston SJ, Mendelson BC. Face lift. Plast Reconstr Surg 2011;128(6):747e–64e.

29. Owsley JQ. Elevation of the malar fat pad superficial to the orbicularis oculi muscle for correction of prominent nasolabial folds. Clin Plast Surg 1995;22:279–93.

30. Mendelson BC. Surgery of the superficial musculoaponeurotic system: principles of release, vectors and fixation. Plast Reconstr Surg 2001;107(6):1545–52.

31. Hamra ST. The deep-plane rhytidectomy. Plast Reconstr Surg 1990;86:53–63.

32. Wong CH, Mendelson BC. Facial Soft-Tissue Spaces and Retaining Ligaments of the Midcheek: Defining the Premaxillary Space. Plast Reconstr Surg 2013;132(1):49–56. https://doi.org/10.1097/PRS.0b013e3182910a57.

33. Mendelson BC & Wong CH. Surgical Anatomy of the Middle Premasseter Space and Its Application in Sub–SMAS Face Lift Surgery.

34. Knize DM. Anatomic concepts for brow lift procedures. Plast Reconstr Surg 2009;124(6):2118–26.

35. Pitanguy I, Ramos AS. The frontal branch of the facial nerve: the importance of its variations in face lifting. Plast Reconstr Surg 1966;38(4):352–6.

36. Pessa JE. An algorithm of facial aging: verification of Lambros's theory by three-dimensional stereolithography, with reference to the pathogenesis of midfacial aging, scleral show, and the lateral suborbital trough deformity. Plast Reconstr Surg 2000;106(2):479–88.

37. Bernstein L, Nelson RH. Surgical anatomy of the extraparotid distribution of the facial nerve. Arch Otolaryngol 1984;110(3):177–83.

38. Furnas DW. Landmarks for the trunks and the temporofacial division of the facial nerve. Br J Surg 1965;52:694–6.

39. Stuzin JM, Wagstrom L, Kawamoto HK, et al. Anatomy of the frontal branch of the facial nerve: the significance of the temporal fat pad. Plast Reconstr Surg 1989;83(2):265–71.

40. Agarwal CA, Mendenhall SD III, Foreman KB, et al. The course of the frontal branch of the facial nerve in relation to fascial planes: an anatomic study. Plast Reconstr Surg 2010;125(2):532–7.

41. Trussler AP, Stephan P, Hatef D, et al. The frontal branch of the facial nerve across the zygomatic arch: anatomical relevance of the high-SMAS technique. Plast Reconstr Surg 2010;125(4):1221–9.

42. Ramirez OM, Santamaria R. Spatial orientation of motor innervation of the lower orbicularis oculi muscle. Aesthet Surg J 2000;20:107.

43. Ruess W, Owsley JQ. The anatomy of the skin and fascial layers of the face in aesthetic surgery. Clin Plast Surg 1987;14(4):677–82.

44. Mendelson BC, Freeman ME, Wu W, et al. Surgical anatomy of the lower face: the premasseter space, the jowl, and the labiomandibular fold. Aesthet Plast Surg 2008;32(2):185–95.

45. Baker DC, Conley J. Avoiding facial nerve injuries in rhytidectomy. Anatomical variations and pitfalls. Plast Reconstr Surg 1979;64(6):781–95.

46. Knize DM. The superficial lateral canthal tendon: anatomic study and clinical application to lateral canthopexy. Plast Reconstr Surg 2002;109(3):1149–57.

47. Ellenbogen R. Pseudo-paralysis of the mandibular branch of the facial nerve after platysmal face-lift operation. Plast Reconstr Surg 1979;63(3):364–8.

48. Salinas NL, Jackson O, Dunham B, et al. Anatomical dissection and modified Sihler stain of the lower branches of the facial nerve. Plast Reconstr Surg 2009;124(6):1905–15.

49. Chowdhry S, Yoder EM, Cooperman RD, et al. Locating the cervical motor branch of the facial nerve: anatomy and clinical application. Plast Reconstr Surg 2010;126(3):875–9.

50. Ozturk CN, Ozturk C, Huettner F, et al. A Failsafe Method to Avoid Injury to the Great Auricular Nerve. Aesthet Surg J 2014;34(1):16–21.

51. McKinney P, Katrana DJ. Prevention of injury to the great auricular nerve during rhytidectomy. Plast Reconstr Surg 1980;66(5):675–9.

52. Singer DP, Sullivan PK. Submandibular gland I: an anatomic evaluation and surgical approach to submandibular gland resection for facial rejuvenation. Plast Reconstr Surg 2003;112(4):1150–4.

53. Auersvald A, Auersvald LA, Oscar Uebel C. Subplatysmal necklift: a retrospective analysis of 504 patients. Aesthet Surg J 2017;37(1):1–11.

54. Larson JD, Tierney WS, Ozturk CN, et al. Defining the fat compartments in the neck: a cadaver study. Aesthet Surg J 2014;34(4):499–506.

55. Ramirez OM. Multidimensional evaluation and surgical approaches to neck rejuvenation. Clin Plast Surg 2014;41(1):99–107.

56. Rohrich RJ, Pessa JE. The anatomy and clinical implications of perioral submuscular fat. Plast Reconstr Surg 2009;124(1):266–71.

57. Charafeddine AH, Couto RA, Zins JE. Neck Rejuvenation: Anatomy and Technique. Clin Plast Surg 2019;46(4):573–86. https://doi.org/10.1016/j.cps.2019.06.004.

58. Pilsl U, Anderhuber F. The chin and adjacent fat compartments. Dermatol Surg 2010;36(2):214–8. https://doi.org/10.1111/j.1524-4725.2009.01424.

59. Mendelson BC, Hartley W, Scott M, et al. Age-related changes of the orbit and mid-cheek and the implications for facial rejuvenation. Aesthet Plast Surg 2007;31(5):419–23.

60. Pessa JE, Garza PA, Love VM, et al. The anatomy of the labiomandibular fold. Plast Reconstr Surg 1998;101(2):482–6. https://doi.org/10.1097/00006534-199802000-00037.

61. Stuzin JM. Restoring facial shape in face lifting: the role of skeletal support in facial analysis and midface soft-tissue repositioning. Plast Reconstr Surg 2007;119(1):362–76.

The Fascias of the Forehead and Temple Aligned—An Anatomic Narrative Review

Fabio Ingallina, MD[a,1], Michael G. Alfertshofer[b,1], Leonie Schelke, MD[c,d], Peter J. Velthuis, MD, PhD[d], Konstantin Frank, MD[b], Samir Mardini, MD[e], Elena Millesi[e], Denis Ehrl, MD, PhD[b], Jeremy B. Green, MD[f], Sebastian Cotofana, MD, PhD[g,*]

KEYWORDS

- Forehead anatomy • Temple anatomy • Frontalis muscle • Facial anatomy • Fascial layers

KEY POINTS

- The 5-layered arrangement of the scalp is continuous with the forehead and the temple. A total of 8 layers can be identified in the forehead and a total of 13 layers in the scalp, which show complex interconnections.
- The layers of the scalp are continuous with the layers of the forehead. Although the other layers of the scalp remain the same in the forehead region, the galea aponeurotica (layer III) of the scalp separates into 3 more layers: suprafrontalis fascia, frontalis muscle, and subfrontalis fascia.
- In the temple, the skin (layer I) and the superficial fatty layer (layer II) are continuous with the scalp. The galea aponeurotica (layer III) separates into 2 laminae (superficial temporal fascia) that enclose the superficial temporal artery. The loose areolar tissue (layer IV) of the scalp forms a separate fascia (innominate fascia) in its superficial aspect, which is overlying the loose areolar tissue of the temple. The periosteum (layer V) of the scalp is continuous with the deep temporal fascia that separates into a superficial and a deep lamina.

INTRODUCTION

In recent years, facial anatomy has received increasing attention because of the rise of minimally-invasive procedures for esthetic purposes.[1,2] These procedures involve neuromodulators or soft tissue fillers injected into the facial soft tissues to ameliorate the signs of aging.[3–6] Facial anatomy, however, has evolved from a 2-dimensional and static understanding into a 3-dimensional (3D) and functional understanding because of the incorporation of novel research methodologies like skin vector displacement analyses,[7] 3D volumetric assessment,[8] skin-surface derived electromyography,[9,10] eye tracking technology,[11–13] and ultrasound imaging.[14–16] The latter allows for the in-vivo real-time visualization of the facial soft tissues, which enables health care professionals to identify subdermal structures without performing surgery or anatomic dissections.

[a] Private Practice, Catania, Italy; [b] Department for Hand, Plastic and Aesthetic Surgery, Ludwig – Maximilian University Munich, Germany; [c] Private Practice, Amsterdam, Netherlands; [d] Department of Dermatology, Erasmus MC, University Medical Centre, Rotterdam, Netherlands; [e] Division of Plastic and Reconstructive Surgery, Mayo Clinic, Rochester, MN 55902, USA; [f] Skin Associates of South Florida and Skin Research Institute, Coral Gables, FL 33146, USA; [g] Department of Clinical Anatomy, Mayo Clinic College of Medicine and Science, Mayo Clinic, Stabile Building 9-38, 200 First Street, Rochester, MN 55905, USA

[1] Both authors contributed equally to this work.

* Corresponding author.

E-mail address: cotofana.sebastian@mayo.edu

Facial Plast Surg Clin N Am 30 (2022) 215–224
https://doi.org/10.1016/j.fsc.2022.01.006
1064-7406/22/© 2022 Elsevier Inc. All rights reserved.

With this new research, the understanding of facial anatomy has evolved to the concept that facial soft tissues are arranged in layers and that those layers are interconnected throughout the face.[17–24] This pan-facial connection of facial layers allows for the development of new treatment strategies like the "temporal lifting technique"[25–27] and the use of soft tissue fillers for lifting the facial soft tissues[8]; this is a different and novel approach, which can be best explained by the underlying anatomy.

The understanding of the layered anatomy of the upper face is crucial when trying to relate the layers of the forehead to the temple and between these two to the layers of the scalp. The clinical relevance of this understanding has recently been demonstrated with the development of the interfascial injection technique for the temple.[26] Here, the layers of the forehead are being used to safely and precisely target the temple for treating temporal hollowing and to influence the appearance of the periorbital area and the midface.[28] This is one example, demonstrating the clinical applicability of advanced anatomic knowledge for best practice and increased patient safety.

However, to date, there is no clear alignment between the anatomic layers of the scalp, forehead, and temple. Therefore, it is the objective of this anatomic narrative review to summarize currently accepted concepts of the layers of the upper face and to align them into a unifying nomenclature and understanding.

MATERIALS AND METHODS

This study is based on a literature review and on the anatomic experience of the authors who have multiple years of experience in cadaveric dissections, facial surgery, and minimally invasive facial procedures.

For the literature review, the PubMed electronic database was screened. Two different search queries were conducted to gather the appropriate articles. The first search focused on the anatomy of the temple and included the following terms: temple AND anatomy OR nomenclature OR layers, temporal fascia AND anatomy OR names OR layers, temporoparietal fascia AND anatomy, temporal AND layer OR anatomy OR flap OR reconstruction OR fascia, temporal layers, tempo* AND fascia AND anatomy, tempo* AND fascia, and temporal region AND layers. The second query identified articles for the forehead. This search was conducted by using the following search terms: forehead AND anatomy OR surgical anatomy OR imaging OR flap OR reconstruction,

forehead AND imaging AND anatomy, galea AND anatomy OR flap or fascia, subgaleal AND anatomy, galea aponeurotica AND anatomy, and scalp AND anatomy OR surgical anatomy. Both queries were limited to English studies that had been conducted in humans. Articles relevant for the temple were limited to the years 2013 to 2021, whereas relevant articles for the forehead had no period limitation. The reason to limit the temple literature search to 2013 was based on a previous literature review.[29] Careful selection was made based on the title and the abstract. Studies were only eligible for inclusion if the anatomic structure of the temple and forehead anatomy were discussed. The remaining articles were excluded if they did not contain information about the layers of one of the aforementioned anatomic regions.

Anatomic descriptions provided herein represent the knowledge and the experience of the authors and should be regarded as such.

RESULTS
Scalp

The term "scalp" can be regarded as an acronym for the 5 parallel layers that can be found in the area of the upper face which is covered by hairs: skin (layer 1), superficial (subdermal) fatty layer (layer 2) (= connective tissue), galea aponeurotica (layer 3) (= aponeurosis), loose areolar tissue (layer 4), and periosteum (layer 5) (**Table 1**).

Most arterial and venous blood supply travel within layer 2 but some arteries can be found in layer 5 as well. Layer 4 is predominantly avascular and can be considered as a safe and feasible dissection plane.

Forehead

The layers of the forehead are continuous with the layers of the scalp. The change in nomenclature occurs anterior to the hairline and is bounded laterally by the temporal crests (= the boundary between forehead and temple) and inferiorly by the superior orbital rim. The following layers can be identified in the forehead: skin (layer 1), superficial (subdermal) fatty layer (layer 2), suprafrontalis fascia (layer 3), frontalis muscle (layer 4), retrofrontalis fat (layer 5), subfrontalis fascia (layer 6), loose areolar tissue in the upper forehead and preperiosteal fat in the lower lateral forehead (layer 7), and periosteum (layer 8) (**Figs. 1–3** and **Table 1**).

Although the skin (layer 1), superficial (subdermal) fatty layer (layer 2), loose areolar tissue (layer 4), and periosteum (layer 5) are continuous between scalp and forehead, the layer 3 structures change and diversify when transitioning into the forehead. The galea aponeurotica separates into 3 layers:

Table 1
Overview of the fascial connections and the numbered layered arrangement of the forehead, scalp, and temple

Layers	Forehead	Scalp	Temple	Layers
1	Skin[30,31]	Skin[31–33]	Skin[26,33]	1
2	Superficial (Subdermal) fatty layer[26]	Superficial (Subdermal) fatty layer[26]	Superficial (Subdermal) fatty layer[26]	2
3	Suprafrontalis fascia[34,35]	Galea aponeurotica[31–33]	Superficial lamina of superficial temporal fascia[36,37]	3
4	Frontalis muscle[30,31]		Deep lamina of superficial temporal fascia[36,37]	4
5	Retrofrontalis fat[34,35]		Deep temporal fat[38,39]	5
6	Subfrontalis fascia[34,35]		Innominate fascia[17,40,41]	6
7	Loose areolar tissue[31,42,43] (in upper forehead) Preperiosteal fat[34,35] (in lower forehead)	Loose areolar tissue[31]	Loose areolar tissue[44–46] (in upper temple)	7
8	Periosteum[30,31]	Periosteum[31–33]	Superficial lamina of deep temporal fascia[26,40,47]	8
			Superficial temporal fat pad[26,40,48]	9
			Deep lamina of deep temporal fascia[26,40,47]	10
			Deep temporal fat pad[26,41,49] (= Temporal extension of buccal fat pad of Bichat)[26,47]	11
			Temporalis muscle[26,33]	12
			Periosteum[26,33]	13

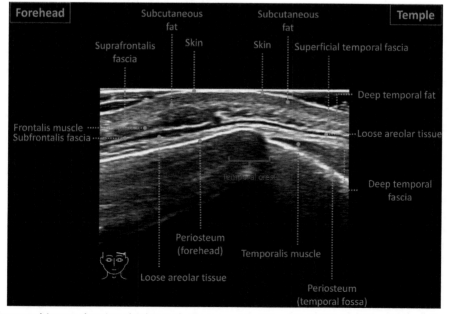

Fig. 1. Ultrasound image showing the layered arrangement of the frontotemporal transition at the temporal crest. Anatomic structures labeled in green indicate structures of the forehead, whereas structures labeled in blue indicate structures of the temple.

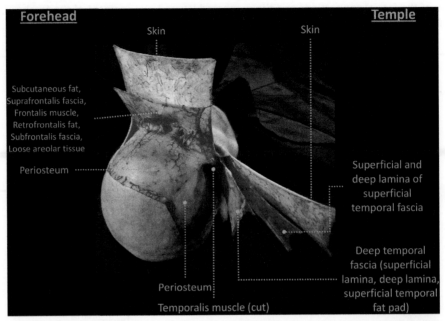

Fig. 2. Cadaveric dissection of the layers of the forehead and temple. Anatomic structures labeled in green indicate structures of the forehead, whereas structures labeled in blue indicate structures of the temple.

suprafrontalis fascia, frontalis muscle, and subfrontalis fascia. Between the frontalis muscle and the subfrontalis fascia, a layer of fat can be identified, which is continuous with the preseptal fat and the retro-orbicularis fat and is termed analogous as retrofrontalis fat (see **Fig. 3**). This fat provides protection and insulation for the deep branch of the supraorbital and supratrochlear arteries and for the branches of the supraorbital and supratrochlear nerve. In the lower lateral forehead, a deep layer of fat can be found in layer 4, which is termed the preperiosteal fat, analogous to the fat within the prezygomatic space in the lateral infraorbital region.

The superficial branches of the supraorbital and supratrochlear arteries travel after they emerge from their respective foraminae superficial to the frontalis muscle but covered by the suprafrontalis fascia and enveloped by the superficial (subdermal) fatty layer. The deep branches travel within the retrofrontalis fat until they change their planes in the upper forehead and travel likewise superficial to the frontalis muscle but deep to the suprafrontalis fascia to connect to the superficial/anterior branch of the superficial temporal artery.

The sensory supraorbital and supratrochlear nerves travel within the retrofrontalis fat initially and become superficial as they accompany the arteries in their change of plane. However, the deep/lateral branch of the supraorbital nerve travels within the periosteum with connections to the subfrontalis fascia and forms in this way the lateral boundary of the deep central forehead compartment or the medial boundary of the deep lateral forehead compartment.

Temple

The layers of the temple are continuous with the layers of the scalp. The change in nomenclature occurs inferior to the hairline and is bounded medially by the temporal crests (= boundary between forehead and temple) and inferiorly by the zygomatic arch. The following layers can be identified in the temple: skin (layer 1), superficial (subdermal) fatty layer (layer 2), superficial lamina of superficial temporal fascia (layer 3), deep lamina of superficial temporal fascia (layer 4), deep temporal fat (layer 5), innominate fascia (layer 6), loose areolar tissue (layer 7), superficial lamina of deep temporal fascia (layer 8), superficial temporal fat pad (layer 9), deep lamina of deep temporal fascia (layer 10), deep temporal fat pad (= temporal extension of the buccal fat pad of Bichat) (layer 11), temporalis muscle (layer 12), and periosteum (layer 13) (see **Figs. 1–3**; **Fig. 4** and **Table 1**).

The skin and the superficial (subdermal) fatty layer are continuous with the scalp. The galea aponeurotica, however, separates into two very thin laminae that enclose the superficial temporal artery on its course toward the forehead and are termed the superficial temporal fascia together. The loose areolar tissue in the scalp forms in its superficial aspect a separate fascia, which is termed in the temple the innominate fascia. This fascia is

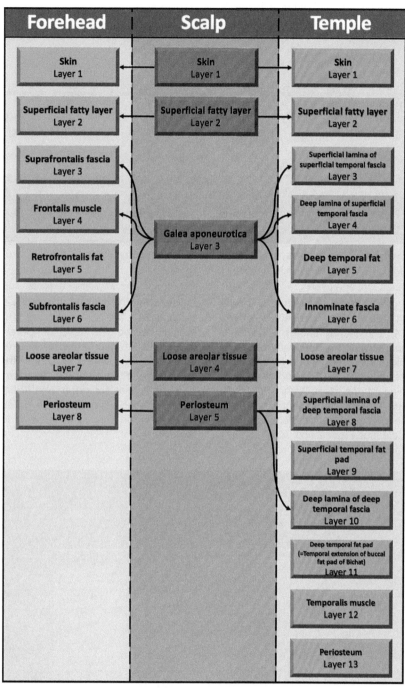

Fig. 3. Schematic diagram showing the layers of the forehead, scalp, and temple. Although only 5 layers can be distinguished in the scalp, the forehead consists of 8 layers and the temple consists of 13 layers. In the forehead, the suprafrontalis fascia (layer 4), frontalis muscle (layer 5), and subfrontalis fascia (layer 7) can be seen as a derivate of the galea aponeurotica (layer 3) of the scalp. In the temple, the superficial and deep lamina of the superficial temporal fascia, as well as the innominate fascia, can be seen as a derivate of the galea aponeurotica (layer 3) of the scalp. In the temple, the superficial and deep lamina of the deep temporal fascia are derived from the periosteum of the scalp, which resembles layer 5.

overlying the loose areolar tissue of the temple and does not extend caudal to the inferior temporal septum. Caudal to the inferior temporal septum, the deep fat of the temple can be found, which is supported by the underlying very thin layer of innominate fascia and loose connective tissue.

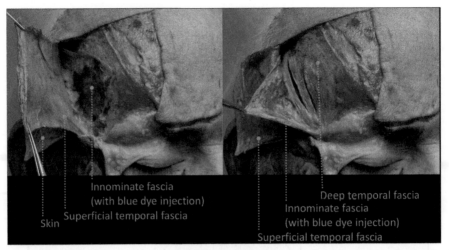

Fig. 4. Cadaveric dissection of the layers in the temple showing the innominate fascia (visualized using blue dye) between the superficial temporal fascia and the deep temporal fascia.

Together they overly the deep temporal fascia which is continuous with the periosteum of the scalp (see **Fig. 4**). The deep temporal fascia separates into a superficial and a deep lamina before their connection to the zygomatic arch and both laminae enclose the superficial temporal fat pad. The deep lamina of the deep temporal fascia covers the deep temporal fat pad (= temporal extension of the buccal fat pad of Bichat) and the temporalis muscle (see **Figs. 2** and **3**).

The frontal branch of the facial nerve travels protected by the deep temporal fat between the superficial and the deep temporal fascia from the temple into the forehead, whereas the middle temporal vein travels between the superficial and the deep lamina of the deep temporal fascia. The superficial temporal and the zygomatico-orbital arteries travel within the superficial temporal fascia and therefore between its 2 laminae (**Fig. 5**).

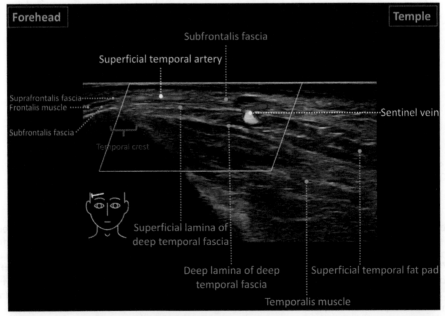

Fig. 5. Ultrasound image showing the superficial temporal artery located within the superficial temporal fascia in the temple and located between the frontalis muscle (deep) and the suprafrontalis fascia (superficial). The middle temporal vein is changing planes after piercing the superficial lamina of the deep temporal fascia and into the loose connective tissue of the temple and later of the forehead.

DISCUSSION

This anatomic narrative review seeks to align the nomenclature of the layered arrangement of the scalp, forehead, and temple. Although these regions have connecting fascial layers, vessels, and nerves, to the authors' knowledge, there is no study to date that aligns the anatomy between those 3 sites, describing how distinct fascial layers are interconnected (see **Fig. 3**).

One of the findings of this narrative review is the diverse nomenclature being used in surgical procedures and anatomic descriptions of the scalp, forehead, and temple throughout the literature. The authors did their best to summarize the literature but might have not included all articles published this far; this can be regarded as a limitation of this study.

It is a novel concept that the galea aponeurotica separates into three different fascial layers when transitioning from the scalp to the forehead but this idea is supported by functional anatomic and clinical reports.[20,50,51] Recently, the line of convergence was introduced into the literature which has greatest clinical relevance for treating horizontal forehead lines with neuromodulators.[52] This horizontal functional line describes a region of the frontalis muscle where its cranial end (= attachment to the galea aponeurotica) and its caudal end (= attachment to the skin of the eyebrow medially and attachment and fusion with the orbicularis oculi muscle laterally) converge during muscular contraction. In this area, no movement of the overlying forehead skin is observed because of the antagonistic movements of the muscle, which is the result of appropriating its caudal and cranial ends. This is only possible when envisioning the frontalis muscle to be encapsulated between two covering fascias comparable to a sleeping bag. The fascia on its superficial surface connects with the overlying skin and allows for proper and direct force transmission corresponding to the muscle contraction status.[34,53,54] This explains why with frontalis muscle contraction the overlying skin forms horizontal wrinkles as opposed to some other facial areas and why the eyebrows move cranially while the hairline moves caudally. These antagonistic movements are possible if there is a strong connection of the muscles' surface and a gliding plane deep to the muscle but separated from the supraperiosteal plane. The presence of a deep fascia = subfrontalis fascia (layer 6) allows for the approximation of the hairline to the eyebrows without compressing the underlying vessels and nerves against the frontal bone.

The anterior branch of the superficial temporal artery emerges from deeper planes 1 cm anterior and 1 cm superior to the apex of the tragus,[26] and travels inside the superficial temporal fascia to reach the forehead. To allow for the coverage of the artery on both sides with a protective fascia, a superficial (layer 3) and a deep (layer 4) lamina is needed. When the artery passes the temporal crest medially, it can be identified superficial to the frontalis muscle.[55] This implies that the superficial lamina of the superficial temporal fascia of the temple (layer 3) is continuous with the suprafrontalis fascia of the forehead (layer 3), whereas the deep lamina of the superficial temporal fascia of the temple (layer 4) is continuous with the frontalis muscle in the forehead (layer 4). This allows for the understanding of the pathway of the artery and the connection between the superficial fascial layers of the forehead and temple (see **Fig. 5**). This is supported by the finding that the superficial temporal fascia is continuous with the orbicularis oculi muscle[17–19] and that this superficially locate muscle is also in direct continuation with the frontalis muscle.[20,21]

The subfrontalis fascia of the forehead is a recently discovered structure and its connection to the temple can be established when accepting the existence of the innominate fascia.[17,18,38,40] The latter was not incorporated in recent descriptions of temporal anatomy but plays an integral role when trying to align the layers of the forehead and temple.[26,56,57] In the forehead, the branches of the supraorbital and supratrochlear nerve travel protected within the retrofrontalis fat which is continuous with the retro-orbicularis oculi fat. Previously, a connection between the forehead and the temple was termed the "superior interval" and described the spatial connection between the inferior temporal compartment and the retro-orbicularis oculi fat.[29] This connection was based on the continuation of a deep layer of fat which protects nerve branches traveling from the temple to the forehead and vice versa (layer 5). As it is known that the frontalis muscle receives its neural supply from deep,[58,59] it is plausible that the frontal branches of the facial nerve travel deep to the frontalis muscle (layer 4) and therefore have to be deep to the deep lamina of the superficial temporal fascia (layer 4) located within the deep fat of the temple.[38,60,61] In the forehead, however, these branches are protected from the supraperiosteal plane by the subfrontalis fascia (layer 6),[38,62] which indicates that this fascial plane has to be deep to the deep fat of the temple. During surgical repair of zygomatic arch fractures, reposition of the arch is performed by approaching the arch deep to the frontal branches of the facial nerve. This is possible due to the presence of a protective layer of fascia and loose areolar tissue. The innominate fascia of the temple continues in the forehead as the subfrontalis fascia and in the scalp as the deep portion of the galea aponeurotica and the connecting interface between the loose areolar tissue and galea.[17,29,63] (see **Fig. 3**).

Previous studies have shown that the middle temporal vein pierces the superficial lamina of the deep temporal fascia lateral to the tail of the eyebrow.[64,65] (see **Fig. 5**) Upon emergence from the deep temporal fascia, the vein does not penetrate the innominate fascia but travels deep to this fascia when reaching the supraorbital region of the forehead. There, the vein can be found deep to the subfrontalis fascia within the preperiosteal fat which is in close relationship to the supraorbital attachment of the orbicularis retaining ligament. Here the vein is termed sentinel vein and connects to the superficial temporal vein close to the auricle.[64] The course of the middle temporal/sentinel vein can be best understood when incorporating the concept of the continuation between the innominate fascia of the temple and the subfrontalis fascia of the forehead; the vein travels deep to this fascia.

Recent advancements in treating temporal hollowing with soft tissue fillers include the interfascial injection technique.[26,28,66] This technique entails injecting the product deep to the superficial temporal fascia and superficial to the deep temporal fascia with periosteal contact of a 22G–25G 50 mm blunt tip cannula of the forehead 1 cm medial and 1 cm inferior to the hairline.[66] After periosteal contact is established in the forehead (layer 8), the cannula is pointed toward the temple and advanced in constant contact with bone. This bony contact is lost lateral to the temporal crest as here the frontal periosteum transitions into the deep temporal fascia of the temple. The blunt tip cannula is gliding on top of the deep temporal fascia, that is, the superficial lamina of the deep temporal fascia (layer 8) when reaching the temple. During product administration, the cannula is deep to the deep temporal fat which includes the motor branches of the facial nerve relevant for the upper facial muscles of expression (layer 5), deep to the innominate fascia (layer 6), but within the loose areolar tissue. This smooth gliding plane allows for homogenous product distribution without risk to the nerve branches. Because the sentinel vein is located in the same plane, care needs to be taken to avoid hematoma formation after accidental injury. Local pressure could help to ameliorate signs and symptoms of sentinel vein injury, and ultrasound follow-up can be performed.

SUMMARY

This anatomic narrative review describes the layered anatomy of the scalp, forehead, and temple and establishes the fascial connections based on literature review, ultrasound imaging, and anatomic dissections. Despite the highly variable nomenclature used for describing fascial layers and their extensions, the anatomy of the 3 upper facial regions can be combined into a unified concept. The 5 layers of the scalp transition into the forehead's 8 layers. In the temple, a total of 13 layers include the innominate fascia as a part of the loose areolar connective tissue. Aligning those anatomic and fascial concepts might allow for the further development of novel surgical and nonsurgical treatment options to enhance outcomes and patient safety.

DISCLOSURE

The authors have nothing to disclose.

REFERENCES

1. ASPS National CLearinghouse of Plastic Surgery Procedural Statistics. Plastic surgery statistics report 2019 2019. https://www.plasticsurgery.org/documents/News/Statistics/2019/plastic-surgery-statistics-full-report-2019.pdf.
2. International Society of Aesthetic Plastic Surgeons. ISAPS international survey on aesthetic/cosmetic procedures performed in 2017 2019. https://www.isaps.org/wp-content/uploads/2019/03/ISAPS_2017_International_Study_Cosmetic_Procedures_NEW.pdf.
3. Sturm LP, Cooter RD, Mutimer KL, et al. A systematic review of dermal fillers for age-related lines and wrinkles. ANZ J Surg 2011;81(1–2):9–17.
4. Burgess CM. Principles of soft tissue augmentation for the aging face. Clin Interv Aging 2006;1(4):349–55. http://www.embase.com/search/resultsbaction=view record&from=export&id=L350325504.
5. Montes JR, Wilson AJ, Chang BL, et al. Technical considerations for filler and neuromodulator refinements. Plast Reconstr Surgery Glob Open 2016; 4(12):e1178. https://doi.org/10.1097/GOX.000000000000001178.
6. Yamauchi PS. Selection and preference for botulinum toxins in the management of photoaging and facial lines: patient and physician considerations. Patient Prefer Adherence 2010;4:345–54.
7. Freytag DL, Alfertshofer MG, Frank K, et al. The difference in facial movement between the medial and the lateral midface: a 3d skin surface vector analysis. Aesthetic Surg J 2021. https://doi.org/10.1093/asj/sjab152.
8. Haidar R, Freytag DL, Frank K, et al. Quantitative analysis of the lifting effect of facial soft-tissue filler injections. Plast Reconstr Surg 2021;147: 765e–76e.

9. Cotofana S, Assemi-Kabir S, Mardini S, et al. Understanding facial muscle aging: a surface electromyography study. Aesthet Surg J 2021;41(9):NP1208–17.

10. Frank K, Moellhoff N, Kaiser A, et al. Signal-to-noise ratio calculations to validate sensor positioning for facial muscle assessment using noninvasive facial electromyography. Facial Plast Surg 2021;37(5):614–24.

11. Frank K, Schuster L, Alfertshofer M, et al. How does wearing a facecover influence the eye movement pattern in times of COVID-19? Aesthet Surg J 2021;41(8):NP1118–24.

12. Pietruski P, Paskal W, Paskal AM, et al. Analysis of the visual perception of female breast aesthetics and symmetry: an eye-tracking study. Plast Reconstr Surg 2019;144(6):1257–66.

13. Dey JK, Ishii LE, Boahene KDO, et al. Measuring outcomes of mohs defect reconstruction using eye-tracking technology. JAMA Facial Plast Surg 2019;21(6):518–25.

14. Frank K, Alfertshofer M, Schenck T, et al. Anatomy of the superior and inferior labial arteries revised: an ultrasound investigation and implication for lip volumization. Aesthet Surg J 2020;40(12):1327–35.

15. Gombolevskiy VA, Gelezhe P, Morozov S, et al. The course of the angular artery in the midface: implications for surgical and minimally invasive procedures. Aesthet Surg J 2020;41(7):805–13.

16. Cotofana S, Alfertshofer M, Frank K, et al. Relationship between vertical glabellar lines and the supratrochlear and supraorbital arteries. Aesthet Surg J. 2020;40(12):1341–8.

17. Accioli de Vasconcellos JJ, Britto JA, Henin D, et al. The fascial planes of the temple and face: an en-bloc anatomical study and a plea for consistency. Br J Plast Surg 2003;56(7):623–9. http://www.ncbi.nlm.nih.gov/pubmed/12969659.

18. Tellioğlu AT, Tekdemir I, Erdemli EA, et al. Temporoparietal fascia: an anatomic and histologic reinvestigation with new potential clinical applications. Plast Reconstr Surg 2000;105(1):40–5.

19. Kang HG, Youn K-H, Kim I-B, et al. Bilayered structure of the superficial facial fascia. Aesthet Surg J 2017;37(6):627–36.

20. Daniel RK, Landon B. Endoscopic forehead lift: anatomic basis. Aesthet Surg J 1997;17(2):97–104.

21. Costin BR, Wyszynski PJ, Rubinstein TJ, et al. Frontalis Muscle Asymmetry and Lateral Landmarks. Ophthal Plast Reconstr Surg 2016;32(1):65–8.

22. Abul-Hassan HS, von Drasek Ascher G, Acland RD. Surgical anatomy and blood supply of the fascial layers of the temporal region. Plast Reconstr Surg 1986;77(1):17–28.

23. Cotofana S, Lachman N. Anatomy of the Facial fat compartments and their relevance in aesthetic surgery. J Dtsch Dermatol Ges 2019;17(4):399–413.

24. Mendelson BC, Jacobson SR. Surgical anatomy of the midcheek: facial layers, spaces, and the midcheek segments. Clin Plast Surg 2008;35(3):395–404.

25. Suwanchinda A, Webb KL, Rudolph C, et al. The posterior temporal supraSMAS minimally invasive lifting technique using soft-tissue fillers. J Cosmet Dermatol 2018;17(4):617–24.

26. Cotofana S, Gaete A, Hernandez CA, et al. The six different injection techniques for the temple relevant for soft tissue filler augmentation procedures – clinical anatomy and danger zones. J Cosmet Dermatol 2020;19(7):1570–9.

27. Hernandez CA, Freytag DL, Gold MH, et al. Clinical validation of the temporal lifting technique using soft tissue fillers. J Cosmet Dermatol 2020;19(10):2529–35.

28. Casabona G, Frank K, Moellhoff N, et al. Full-face effects of temporal volumizing and temporal lifting techniques. J Cosmet Dermatol 2020;19(11):2830–7.

29. O'Brien JX, Ashton MW, Rozen WM, et al. New perspectives on the surgical anatomy and nomenclature of the temporal region. Plast Reconstr Surg 2013;131(3):510–22.

30. Cotofana S, Mian A, Sykes JM, et al. An update on the anatomy of the forehead compartments. Plast Reconstr Surg 2017;139(4):864e–72e.

31. Garritano FG, Quatela VC. Surgical anatomy of the upper face and forehead. Facial Plast Surg 2018;34(2):109–13.

32. Temple CLF, Ross DC. Scalp and forehead reconstruction. Clin Plast Surg 2005;32(3):377–90. vi-vii.

33. Dedhia R, Luu Q. Scalp reconstruction. Curr Opin Otolaryngol Head Neck Surg 2015;23(5):407–14.

34. Cotofana S, Velthuis PJ, Alfertshofer M, et al. The change of plane of the supratrochlear and supraorbital arteries in the forehead - an ultrasound-based investigation. Aesthet Surg J. 2021;41(11):NP1589–98.

35. Davidovic K, Melnikov DV, Frank K, et al. To click or not to click – The importance of understanding the layers of the forehead when injecting neuromodulators – A clinical, prospective, interventional, split-face study. J Cosmet Dermatol 2020;20(5):1385–92.

36. Beheiry EE, Abdel-Hamid FAM. An anatomical study of the temporal fascia and related temporal pads of fat. Plast Reconstr Surg 2007;119(1):136–44.

37. Jiang P, Chen Q, Huang W. [An anatomy study of temporal layers : the safe space for hyaluronic acid injection]. Zhonghua Zheng Xing Wai Ke Za Zhi 2016;32(4):280–5.

38. Agarwal CA, Mendenhall SD, Foreman KB, et al. The course of the frontal branch of the facial nerve in relation to fascial planes: An anatomic study. Plast Reconstr Surg 2010;125(2):532–7.

39. Pankratz J, Baer J, Mayer C, et al. Depth transitions of the frontal branch of the facial nerveimplications in smas rhytidectomy. JPRAS Open 2020;26:102–8.

40. Chi D, Kim JH, Kim TK, et al. Cadaveric study of deep temporal fascia for autologous rhinoplasty grafts: Dimensions of the temporal compartment in Asians. Arch Plast Surg 2020;47(6):604–12.

41. Vaca EE, Purnell CA, Gosain AK, et al. Postoperative temporal hollowing: is there a surgical approach that prevents this complication? A systematic review and anatomic illustration. J Plast Reconstr Aesthet Surg 2017;70(3):401–15.

42. Ridgway JM, Larrabee WF. Anatomy for blepharoplasty and brow-lift. Facial Plast Surg 2010;26(3): 177–85.

43. Sharman AM, Kirmi O, Anslow P. Imaging of the skin, subcutis, and galea aponeurotica. Semin Ultrasound CT MR 2009;30(6):452–64.

44. Sykes JM, Riedler KL, Cotofana S, et al. Superficial and deep facial anatomy and its implications for rhytidectomy. Facial Plast Surg Clin North Am 2020; 28(3):243–51.

45. Jaquet Y, Higgins KM, Enepekides DJ. The temporoparietal fascia flap: a versatile tool in head and neck reconstruction. Curr Opin Otolaryngol Head Neck Surg 2011;19(4):235–41.

46. Breithaupt AD, Jones DH, Braz A, et al. Anatomical basis for safe and effective volumization of the temple. Dermatol Surg 2015;41(Suppl 1):S278–83.

47. Idone F, Bolletta E, Piedimonte A, et al. Temporal fossa atrophy in aesthetic medicine: anatomy, classification, and treatment. Plast Reconstr Surgery Glob Open 2020;8(10):e3169.

48. Huang RL, Xie Y, Wang W, et al. Anatomical study of temporal fat compartments and its clinical application for temporal fat grafting. Aesthet Surg J 2017; 37(8):855–62.

49. Li H, Li K, Jia W, et al. Does the deep layer of the deep temporalis fascia really exist? J Oral Maxillofac Surg 2018;76(8):1824.e1–7.

50. Grosshans E, Fersing J, Marescaux J. [Subaponeurotic lipoma of the forehead]. Ann Dermatol Venereol 1987;114(3):335–40.

51. Brass D, Oliphant TJ, McHanwell S, et al. Successful treatment of forehead lipoma depends on knowledge of the surgical anatomy: a step-by-step guide. Clin Exp Dermatol 2016;41(1):3–7.

52. Cotofana S, Freytag DL, Frank K, et al. The bidirectional movement of the frontalis muscle - introducing the line of convergence and its potential clinical relevance. Plast Reconstr Surg 2020; 145(5):1155–62.

53. Knize DM. An anatomically based study of the mechanism of eyebrow ptosis. Plast Reconstr Surg 1996;97(7):1321–33.

54. Sandulescu T, Franzmann M, Jast J, et al. Facial fold and crease development: a new morphological approach and classification. Clin Anat 2019;32(4): 573–84.

55. Jo YW, Hwang K, Huan F, et al. Perforating frontal branch of the superficial temporal artery as related to subcutaneous forehead lift. J Craniofac Surg 2012;23(6):1861–3.

56. Freytag DL, Frank K, Haidar R, et al. Facial safe zones for soft tissue filler injections: a practical guide. J Drugs Dermatol 2019;18(9):896–902.

57. Pavicic T, Minokadeh A, Cotofana S. The temple and forehead. In: Inject fill facial shap contouring. 2019. p. 63–76. https://doi.org/10.1002/9781119046974. ch3.

58. Fatah MF. Innervation and functional reconstruction of the forehead. Br J Plast Surg 1991;44(5):351–8. https://doi.org/10.1016/0007-1226(91)90148-D.

59. Hotta TA. Understanding the anatomy of the upper face when providing aesthetic injection treatments. Plast Surg Nurs 2016;36(3):104–9.

60. Stuzin JM, Wagstrom L, Kawamoto HK, et al. Anatomy of the frontal branch of the facial nerve: the significance of the temporal fat pad. Plast Reconstr Surg 1989;83(2):265–71.

61. Sihag RK, Gupta SK, Sahni D, et al. Frontotemporal branch of the facial nerve and fascial layers in the temporal region: a cadaveric study to define a safe dissection plane. Neurol India 2020;68(6):1313–20.

62. Pankratz J, Baer J, Mayer C, et al. Depth transitions of the frontal branch of the facial nerve: implications in SMAS rhytidectomy. JPRAS Open 2020;26:101–8.

63. Tolhurst DE, Carstens MH, Greco RJ, et al. The surgical anatomy of the scalp. Plast Reconstr Surg 1991;87(4):603–4.

64. Yano T, Okazaki M, Yamaguchi K, et al. Anatomy of the middle temporal vein: Implications for skull-base and craniofacial reconstruction using free flaps. Plast Reconstr Surg 2014;134(1):92e–101e.

65. Beer JI, Sieber DA, Scheuer JF 3rd, et al. three-dimensional facial anatomy: structure and function as it relates to injectable neuromodulators and soft tissue fillers. Published online. Plast Reconstr Surgery Glob Open 2016;4(12):e1175.

66. Ingallina F. Faciala anatomy & volumizing injections - superior & middle third - anatomy in 3D aging & aesthetic analysis – advanced techniques of injections. 2017.

Electrophysiologic Frontalis Muscle Response Following Neuromodulator Injections

Konstantin Frank, MD[a,1], Shirin Assemi-Kabir, DDS[a,1],
Michael G. Alfertshofer[a], Denis Ehrl, MD, PhD[a], Robert H. Gotkin, MD, FACS[b],
Nicholas Moellhoff, MD[a], Paul Z. Lorenc, MD[b], Tatjana Pavicic, MD[c],
Claudia A. Hernandez, MD[d], Sebastian Cotofana, MD, PhD[e,*]

KEYWORDS

- Neuromodulators • Facial muscles • Surface electromyography • Motor-unit action potential
- Facial anatomy

KEY POINTS

- This study investigated, for the first time in literature, the relationship between the underlying frontalis muscle activity and overlying forehead skin movement by using sEMG and skin vector displacement analyses.
- Results revealed that a decrease in frontalis muscle MUAP using 25 IU of Incobotulinumtoxin by 20% results in a clinically relevant reduction of forehead line severityA 33% reduction in frontalis muscle MUAP is required to induce a statistically relevant reduction in objectively measured forehead skin movement.

INTRODUCTION

According to the annual statistics conducted by The Aesthetic Society in 2020, a total of 2,643,366 neuromodulator injections were performed in the United States; this generated a revenue of more than 1 billion USD.[1] Most of these procedures involved treatment of the upper face, as it has been shown that the gaze pattern, as well as the focus of attention, shifted toward the upper face owing to face-covering guidelines in times of the pandemic.[2] Upper face neuromodulator injections typically treat the periorbital muscles for lateral canthal lines,[3,4] glabellar muscles for glabellar lines,[5] and the frontalis muscle for horizontal forehead lines.[6–8]

The administered neuromodulator induces a temporary paresis/paralysis of the targeted muscle, which decreases the muscle's ability to contract. The limited contractility of the muscle results in reduced dynamic and static wrinkle

K.F., S.A.-K., M.A., N.M.,C.H and S.C. performed the research. S.C., P.Z.L., T.P., and D.E. designed the research study. R.H.G. and S.C. contributed essential reagents or tools. S.C., S.A.-K., and K.F. analyzed the data. S.C., S.A.-K., and K.F. wrote the paper.
Funding: This study was financially supported by a grant from Merz North America Inc under the grant number 2262019.
[a] Department for Hand, Plastic and Aesthetic Surgery, Ludwig–Maximilian University Munich, Germany; [b] Private Practice, New York, NY, USA; [c] Private Practice, Munich, Germany; [d] CH Dermatologia, Medellin, Colombia; [e] Department of Clinical Anatomy, Mayo Clinic College of Medicine and Science, Mayo Clinic, Stabile Building 9-38, 200 First Street, Rochester, MN 55905, USA
[1] Authors contributed equally.
* Corresponding author. Department of Clinical Anatomy, Mayo Clinic College of Medicine and Science, Mayo Clinic, Stabile Building 9-38, 200 First Street, Rochester, MN 55905.
E-mail address: cotofana.sebastian@mayo.edu

formation of the overlying skin; this is the desired effect of the treatment.

The formation of wrinkles, such as horizontal forehead lines, requires a direct connection between the underlying muscle and the overlying skin. This mandates a network of stable connective tissue adhesions allowing the transmission of muscular contractions to the subdermal interface. This transmission is facilitated in the forehead by the suprafrontalis fascia[9,10] and its subdermal fibrous architecture,[11] which is comparable to the midfacial SMAS (superficial musculo-aponeurotic system).[12] However, with increased skin laxity and/or increased thickness of subcutaneous fat, a direct force transmission can be altered and, despite proper muscular contractions, the overlying skin might not move correspondingly to the contractions of the underlying frontalis muscle. It could also be speculated that a certain degree of muscular movement is necessary to effect movement of the overlying skin; this is of clinical relevance during neuromodulator treatments.

To investigate the influence of frontalis muscle activity on forehead skin movement, this experimental study was designed. To analyze frontalis muscle activity, surface-derived noninvasive electromyography (sEMG) was used, and to measure forehead skin movement, skin vector displacement was derived from surface 3-dimensional (3D) imaging. No study to date combined these 2 methods to evaluate the relationship between muscle contraction and overlying skin movement. It is hoped that this investigation will provide greater clarity on the effects of neuromodulator treatments and will ultimately help to increase efficacy for aesthetic patients seeking neuromodulator injections.

MATERIALS AND METHODS
Study Sample

This interventional study investigated the electrophysiologic response of the frontalis muscle following neuromodulator injections in a total of 11 healthy neuromodulator-naïve volunteers (5 men, 6 women). Study participants were consecutive patients recruited by the Department for Hand, Plastic and Aesthetic Surgery, Ludwig–Maximilian University, Munich, Germany with a mean age of 26.64 (2.0) years (range: 24–30), and a mean body mass index (BMI) of 22.28 (2.0) kg/m^2 (range: 19.0–25.6). Patients were eligible for this study if they had no previous neuromodulator treatments to their forehead or periorbital region and had no previous facial trauma or surgery that could potentially disrupt the integrity of their upper facial anatomy or normal frontalis muscle function.

Written informed consent was obtained from all participants before inclusion in the study for the use of their images and personal data for research purposes. This study was performed in adherence to the Declaration of Helsinki (1996)[13] and received institutional review board approval from REDACTE under the approval number: REDACTED.

Injection Procedure

Study participants were treated for their horizontal forehead lines at the beginning of the study. The following injection pattern was used: a total of 10 injection locations, 2.5 IU each, 5 of which were administered in the upper row located above the line of convergence,[6] and 5 of which were administered in the lower row, that is, below the line of convergence (**Fig. 1**). A total of 25 IU of Incobotulinumtoxin type A (Xeomin, Bocouture; Merz Pharmaceuticals GmbH, Frankfurt am Main, Germany) were administered to each study participant (see **Fig. 1**).

Measurements Conducted

Forehead line severity
Forehead line severity was assessed via a validated 5-point scale (grade 0 = no lines; grade 1 = mild lines; grade 2 = moderate lines; grade 3 = severe lines; grade 4 = very severe lines).[14] Assessment was conducted by an independent observer based on 3D images at rest and during maximal frontalis muscle contraction for each follow-up visit.

Surface-derived noninvasive electromyography
sEMG measurements were conducted consistently and for all study participants following a previously published protocol.[15,16] In brief, 2 noninvasive, surface adherent, wireless sensors were positioned on the forehead of each study participant located 2 cm cranial to the upper margin of the hairy eyebrow in the left and right vertical midpupillary lines.

Study participants were asked to maximally contract their frontalis muscle and elevate their brows 3 times in a row, and the sEMG sensors detected the motor unit action potential (MUAP) of the underlying frontalis muscle for each movement and transmitted the information to the sEMG receiver box (Avanti Trigno Quattro; Delsys Inc, Natick, MA, USA) as described previously.[15,16] The detected MUAP was imported into the proprietary software (EMGworks; Delsys Inc) and analyzed for the variables of interest.

Three-dimensional surface scanning
The skin surface of the forehead of each study participant was captured at rest and during

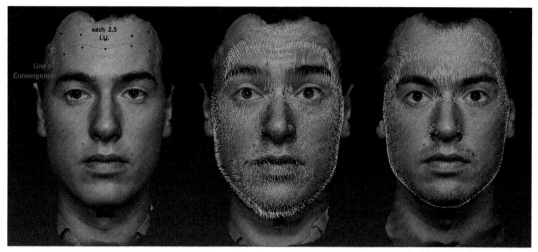

Fig. 1. Injection points in relation to the line of convergence exemplified on a male 26-year-old study participant. Each injection point administered 2.5 IU of Incobotulinumtoxin type A for a total dosage of 25 IU per study participant. (*left*) 3D image of a 26-year-old male study participant showing skin vector displacement during maximal frontalis muscle contraction at baseline (*middle*) and 4 days after the injection procedure (*right*).

maximal frontalis muscle contraction via a 3D camera (Vectra H2, Canfield Scientific Inc, Fairfield, NJ, USA). Differences in skin position between maximal brow elevation and at rest were analyzed using skin vector displacement analysis via the automated algorithm of the Vectra Software Suite as described previously.[17] All measurements were conducted by the same investigator (S.A.-K.) to assure consistency throughout the analyses (see **Fig. 1**).

Analytical Procedure

The variables of interest were the mean value of the 3 performed frontalis muscle contractions calculated as the root-mean-square of the maximal muscle contraction (the signal, in μV) and the root-mean-square of the respective muscle activity at rest (the baseline noise, in μV). The signal-to-noise ratio (SNR) was calculated by using the 20 log function of the ratio between the signal divided by the baseline noise according to the manufacturer's guideline as described previously.[18] The mean values of the left and the right frontalis muscle MUAP were averaged and used for further statistical analyses without side-difference comparisons.

3D skin surface imaging measured the displacement of the forehead skin in a vertical direction comparable to the movement along the y-axis in a Cartesian coordinate system. Values are given in millimeters and represent the difference in skin movement between the resting and maximally contracted forehead skin.

All measurements were conducted before the neuromodulator injections and repeated at days

1, 2, 3, 4, 5, 7, and 14 and at 1, 2, and 4 months following the initial injection procedure.

Differences between genders were calculated using nonparametric Mann-Whitney *U* test, and differences between follow-up time points were calculated using Kruskall-Wallis test. All calculations were performed with IBM SPSS Version 27 (IBM Corp, Armonk, NY, USA), and results were considered statistically significant at a probability level of $P \leq .05$.

RESULTS
General Description

Of the 11 study participants, 100% completed the follow-up period. Men were identified to have an overall statistically significant increase in SNR compared with women with 7.32 (2.3) versus 6.06 (2.6) ($P = .005$), and men were also identified to have an overall greater vertical movement of their forehead skin compared with women with 7.23 (2.4) mm versus 4.82 (1.7) mm ($P<.001$).

Relating the SNR to the respective skin movement, it was revealed that the higher the SNR, the more vertical skin displacement was observed: $r_p = .406$ with $P<.001$, which remained statistically relevant even after gender stratification.

Forehead Line Severity

The median forehead line severity score during maximal frontalis muscle contraction at baseline was 2 (0–4, best to worst) with an interquartile range of 2. At day 2, a statistically significant decrease in forehead line severity was observed to a median score of 1 (2) with $P = .047$, and this

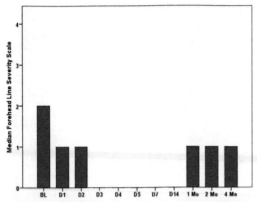

Fig. 2. The median forehead line severity scale (grade 0 = no lines; grade 1 = mild lines; grade 2 = moderate lines; grade 3 = severe lines; grade 4 = very severe lines)[14] evaluated during maximal frontalis muscle contraction at baseline and at each follow-up visit.

was maintained until 1 month after the initial treatment. At 2 months following the initial injection, forehead line severity revealed no statistically significant difference when compared with the baseline value (**Fig. 2**).

Surface-Derived Noninvasive Electromyography

The average SNR at baseline (independent of gender) was 8.45 (3.8) and decreased following the neuromodulator injection across all time points with $P = .003$. The maximal decrease in SNR was observed at 14 days following the treatment with 4.43 and $P = .028$, indicating a decrease of 47.6% when compared with the baseline value (**Fig. 3**).

Three-Dimensional Surface Scanning

The average vertical skin displacement at baseline (independent of gender) was 7.45 (1.9) mm and

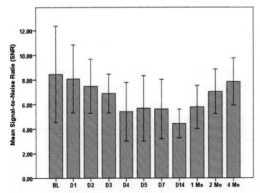

Fig. 3. The mean SNR at each follow-up visit. Error bars indicate ± standard deviation.

decreased at 4 days following the injection to a statistically significant level with 5.43 (2.7) mm and $P = .034$; this indicates a reduction of 27.1% when compared with baseline. This decrease was maintained until 1 month following the treatment and increased in the measurements conducted afterward (**Figs. 4 and 5**).

DISCUSSION

This study investigated, for the first time in the literature, the relationship between underlying frontalis muscle activity and overlying forehead skin movement by using sEMG and skin vector displacement analyses. Using both modalities in a combined study protocol enables one to draw conclusions about the frontalis muscle activity required to move the overlying skin and, in addition, to monitor the direct effect of neuromodulator injections. The decision to include both modalities into 1 study design is based on the biomechanical concept that underlies skin wrinkle formation. The underlying muscle has a certain degree of contractility, which is transmitted to the overlying skin. This force transmission between the muscle and overlying skin is facilitated by a system of connective tissue fibers and fasciae; in the forehead, this is the suprafrontalis fascia[9,10] and its respective subdermal fibrous architecture.[11] This system, however, is also a weak point during force transmission because alterations to this link can influence the movement of the overlying skin and mask the underlying muscle activity. Therefore, the movement of skin and the respective formation of wrinkles are a reflection of an intact connective tissue apparatus and muscle contractility.

This concept influenced patient selection because only healthy, young, and toxin-naïve participants were selected with a mean age of 26.64 (2.0) years (range: 24–30) and a mean BMI of 22.28 (2.0) kg/m^2 (range: 19.0–25.6). This assured that no age-related laxity of the skin or the connective tissue apparatus or weight-related influence on the subdermal fatty layer thickness would influence the force transmission between muscle and skin.

The results of the analyses revealed that neuromodulator injections were effective in reducing forehead line severity starting at day 2 following the treatment and extending until the end of the study observational period. A longer follow-up period would have been able to capture the total duration of the treatment, and future studies will need to address this limitation.

Analyzing the movement of forehead skin with skin vector displacement analyses revealed that the administration of 25 IU of Incobotulinumtoxin

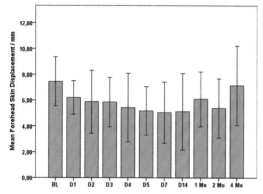

Fig. 4. The mean vertical skin vector displacement at each follow-up visit. Error bars indicate ± standard deviation.

type A to each study participant with a similar injection technique resulted in a maximal decrease of forehead skin movement by 32.2% when compared with the movement amplitude before the treatment. The reduction in movement reached a statistically relevant level between day 4 and day 14 of the follow-up period only and returned to almost pretreatment values toward the end of the observational period. Interestingly, at no point in the follow-up period was the movement of the forehead absent, blocked, or comparable to a "frozen forehead," owing to the injection technique and dosage used. It can be assumed that a higher neuromodulator dose or more injection points would have resulted in a greater reduction of forehead skin movement. However, this clinical study used recently suggested injection points respecting the line of convergence[6] and the administration of the product into the deep plane[8]; this has the aim of wrinkle reduction without affecting eyebrow position or being at risk to cause

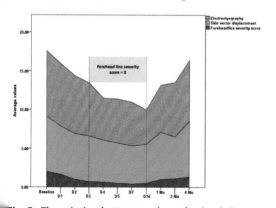

Fig. 5. The relation between values obtained via measurements from electromyography, skin vector displacement, and semiquantitative scoring of forehead line severity during maximal frontalis muscle contraction. Note that the clinically visible effect is ranging between day 3 and 1 month.

lateral hyperelevation ("Spock eyebrow"), or upper eyelid ptosis.

The administration of neuromodulators resulted in the reduction of the MUAP, measured by the SNR, which reached its maximum 14 days following the treatment; this was observed in both men and women. Again, and comparable to the forehead skin movement analyses, the treatment did not eliminate all MUAP. This can possibly be explained by the number of units used and the injection technique used. Future studies will need to address this limitation and expand on the methodology presented herein.

One of the most important findings of this study is the sequence of the detected neuromodulator effects: reduction in semiquantitatively assessed forehead line severity starting at day 3, reduction in objectively assessed forehead skin movement starting at day 4, and reduction in frontalis muscle MUAP having its maximum at day 14 (see **Fig. 5**). This sequence provides a good reflection on the methodology applied. The semiquantitative scoring evaluates the formation of wrinkles and their severity, but the authors' results show that, despite reducing wrinkle severity to a clinically relevant level, skin mobility was still present. This is plausible when analyzing on the biomechanics of wrinkle formation in which a certain degree of skin movement is necessary to approach dermal adhesion points enough to form a bulging between them. Starting at day 3 following the treatment, a reduction of 21.3% in skin movement was sufficient to reduce the forehead line severity from score 2 to 0. This was consistent with the observation at the 1-month follow-up, where skin movement increased again to 18.3%, which resulted in a concomitant increase of forehead line severity from a score of 0 to 1. At day 3, the sEMG revealed that SNR was reduced by 18.6% (compared with baseline), but clinically the forehead line severity reached a score of 0. This indicates that the magnitude in frontalis muscle MUAP reduction is sufficient to achieve a wrinkle severity score of 0 and, therefore, a clinically visible change.

To achieve a statistically significant reduction in objectively assessed forehead skin movement, as observed between day 4 and 14, a reduction of frontalis muscle MUAP of 32.9% or higher is needed. This is novel and interesting, as the authors' results indicate that there is still muscle activity present despite not being reflected on the skin surface. Based on these results, it can be hypothesized that a reduction of up to approximately 30% in SNR of the frontalis muscle's MUAP can be present and still have sufficient contractility to move the overlying skin on a detectable level. Moreover, a reduction of approximately 20% or more can result in a clinically meaningful reduction (here: from score 2–0) in forehead line severity.

This study is not free of limitations. It must be emphasized that the sEMG and the skin vector displacement measurements are summative measurements and include larger areas than only the area where the toxin was administered. For the sEMG measurements, only 1 sensor was used per forehead side, and it can be speculated that the other parts of the frontalis muscle (lower or lateral frontalis) still generate a sufficient signal to alter the locally captured MUAP. For the displacement measures, the measured area was located between the hairline and the upper margin of the eyebrows. As the injection technique was designed to not significantly affect the lower forehead, a certain degree of movement can be expected from this area and thus to influence the summative skin vector analysis. Another limitation of this study is the small sample size. A larger sample would have strengthened the observations, but because of the intense follow-up schedule required, a limited number of volunteers was available. Future studies will need to address this limitation and additionally include other neuromodulators to test their effects on frontalis muscle activity.

SUMMARY

This study investigated, for the first time in literature, the relationship between the underlying frontalis muscle activity and overlying forehead skin movement by using sEMG and skin vector displacement analyses. The results revealed that a decrease in frontalis muscle MUAP using 25 IU of Incobotulinumtoxin by 20% results in a clinically relevant reduction of forehead line severity. At least a 33% reduction in frontalis muscle MUAP is required to induce a statistically relevant reduction in objectively measured forehead skin movement. These results are novel and will help the aesthetic community to better understand neuromodulator effects on the frontalis muscle.

CLINICS CARE POINTS

- Surface Electromyography (sEMG) is a novel technique to evaluate the effect of neurotoxins on the neuromuscular activity of the frontalis muscle.
- The MUAP of the frontalis muscle should be reduced by a third to see a relevant reduction in objectively measured forehead skin movement.

DISCLOSURE

The authors declare no potential conflicts of interest with respect to the research, authorship, and publication of this article.

REFERENCES

1. The American Society for Aesthetic Plastic Surgery. Cosmetic (Aesthetic) Surgery National Data Bank Statistics. 2020. Available at: https://www.surgery.org/sites/default/files/ASAPS-Stats2020_0.pdf. Accessed May 17th, 2021.
2. Frank K, Schuster L, Alfertshofer M, et al. How does wearing a facecover influence the eye movement pattern in times of COVID-19? Aesthet Surg J 2021. https://doi.org/10.1093/asj/sjab121.
3. Kane MAC. Classification of crow's feet patterns among Caucasian women: the key to individualizing treatment. Plast Reconstr Surg 2003;112(5 Suppl): 33S–9S.
4. Brin MF, Boodhoo TI, Pogoda JM, et al. Safety and tolerability of onabotulinumtoxinA in the treatment of facial lines: a meta-analysis of individual patient data from global clinical registration studies in 1678 participants. J Am Acad Dermatol 2009;61(6). https://doi.org/10.1016/j.jaad.2009.06.040.
5. Cotofana S, Pedraza AP, Kaufman J, et al. Respecting upper facial anatomy for treating the glabella with neuromodulators to avoid medial brow ptosis—a refined 3-point injection technique. J Cosmet Dermatol 2021. https://doi.org/10.1111/jocd.14133.
6. Cotofana S, Freytag DL, Frank K, et al. The bidirectional movement of the frontalis muscle - introducing the line of convergence and its potential clinical relevance. Plast Reconstr Surg 2020;145(5): 1155–62.
7. Frank K, Freytag DL, Schenck TL, et al. Relationship between forehead motion and the shape of forehead lines-a 3D skin displacement vector analysis. J Cosmet Dermatol 2019;18(5):1224–9.
8. Davidovic K, Melnikov DV, Frank K, et al. To click or not to click – the importance of understanding the layers of the forehead when injecting neuromodulators – a clinical, prospective, interventional, split-face study. J Cosmet Dermatol 2020. https://doi.org/10.1111/jocd.13875.
9. Cotofana S, Velthuis PJ, Alfertshofer M, et al. The change of plane of the supratrochlear and supraorbital arteries in the forehead—an ultrasound-based investigation. Aesthet Surg J 2021. https://doi.org/10.1093/asj/sjaa421.
10. Knize DM. An anatomically based study of the mechanism of eyebrow ptosis. Plast Reconstr Surg 1996;97(7):1321–33.

11. Sandulescu T, Franzmann M, Jast J, et al. Facial fold and crease development: a new morphological approach and classification. Clin Anat 2019;32(4): 573–84.

12. Sandulescu T, Weniger J, Philippou S, et al. Immunohistochemical evidence of striated muscle cells within midfacial superficial musculoaponeurotic system. Ann Anat 2021;234. https://doi.org/10.1016/j.aanat.2020.151647.

13. WMA Declaration of Helsinki – ethical principles for medical research involving human subjects – WMA – the World Medical Association. Available at: https://www.wma.net/policies-post/wma-declaration-of-helsinki-ethical-principles-for-medical-research-involving-human-subjects/. Accessed August 5, 2018.

14. Flynn TC, Carruthers A, Carruthers J, et al. Validated assessment scales for the upper face. Dermatol Surg 2012;38(2ptII):309–19.

15. Frank K, Möllhoff N, Kaiser A, et al. Optimal positioning of EMG - electrodes in facial muscle assessment. Plast Reconstr Surg 2020.

16. Cotofana S, Assemi-Kabir S, Mardini S, et al. Understanding facial muscle aging: a surface electromyography study. Aesthet Surg J 2021. https://doi.org/10.1093/asj/sjab202.

17. Haidar R, Freytag MDDL, Frank K, et al. Quantitative analysis of the lifting effect of facial soft-tissue filler injections. Plast Reconstr Surg 2021;147(5): 765e–76e.

18. Frank K, Moellhoff N, Giunta R, et al. Signal-to-noise ratio calculations to validate sensor positioning for facial muscle assessment using non-invasive facial electromyography. Facial Plast Surg 2021;37(5): 614–24.

Understanding the Vascular Anatomy of the Face: Introducing the X-Y-Z-Concept

Jonathan M. Sykes, MD[a],*, Haley N. Bray, MD[b],1

KEYWORDS

- Injectable fillers • Complications • Vasculature • Facial anatomy

KEY POINTS

- Vascular compromise is a known devastating complication of injectable fillers.
- Understanding facial anatomy in a layered concept can provide a better understanding of how to avoid vascular injury with injectable fillers.
- The facial vascular anatomy is most predictable in the depth at which it courses in relation to the layers of the face.

INTRODUCTION

The demand for injectable fillers to volumize and rejuvenate the face is increasing. To safely and effectively perform surgery or inject neuromodulators and fillers, the practitioner must have a thorough knowledge of surface anatomy and the structures which lie beneath the skin surface.

As more practitioners enter aesthetic medicine and more varieties of facial fillers emerge, the increased utility of facial fillers to improve both facial aging and facial structure has evolved. The ongoing media blitz of youth and beauty and the constant exposure by media make individuals prioritize facial youth and beauty.

Injectors have realized the power of facial fillers as a versatile solution to improve facial volume and to enhance facial structure. As the demand for facial fillers has increased, so has the frequency and severity of complications related to these injections. The most dreaded complication caused by filler injections is vascular compromise. Intravascular injection of filler and resultant embolism can result in skin discoloration, skin necrosis, and even blindness.

To successfully perform injections and to avoid vascular complications, the practitioner must understand the variant facial anatomy. Thorough knowledge of the layered anatomy allows the practitioner to apply techniques that avoid intravascular injection and their associated vascular complications.

THE LAYERS OF THE FACE

Although a few exceptions exist, the skin, subcutaneous tissues, and superficial and deep fascial layers of the face are consistent in their relationships and can be designated with a common numbering system. These layers can be numbered I–V. Although the names of the individual layers differ in various regions of the forehead, temple, face, and neck, the relative relationships of these layers remain constant. The muscles, nerves, and vascular structures, however, vary in their position and relationship to the layers.

The skin, subcutaneous tissues, and superficial and deep fascial layers of the face are consistent in their relationships and can be designated with a common numbering system. These layers can

a Department of Facial Plastic & Reconstructive Surgery, University of California Davis, Sacramento, CA, USA;
b Department of Otolaryngology-Head and Neck Surgery, Saint Louis University School of Medicine, St Louis, MO, USA
1 Present address: 1298 Antelope Creek Drive Apt 214, Roseville, CA 95678.
* Corresponding author. Department of Facial Plastic & Reconstructive Surgery, University of California Davis, 3301 C Street, 2221 Stockton Blvd Suite 1100, Sacramento, CA 95817.
E-mail address: jmsykes@ucdavis.edu

Facial Plast Surg Clin N Am 30 (2022) 233–237
https://doi.org/10.1016/j.fsc.2022.01.013
1064-7406/22/© 2022 Published by Elsevier Inc.

Table 1 Simplified arrangement of the layers of the face	
I	Skin
II	Subcutaneous tissue/superficial fat
III	Superficial fascia
IV	Loose areolar tissue/deep fat
V	Deep fascia/Periosteum

be numbered I–V, with each layer being consistent in tissue type throughout different regions of the face. This layered designation is shown in **Table 1**.

The thickness of tissue layers differs in different facial regions, but the relationship between layers is consistent. The attachment of the skin (layer I) to the superficial fascia (layer III) is tightly adherent, while the connections between the superficial fascia (layer III) and the deep fascia (layer V) are relatively loose.

The various facial layers are connected by facial ligaments. The facial ligaments are condensations of connective tissue which subdivide the face into compartments and connect the facial layers from the skin superficially to the bone deeply. The ligaments can be termed true, which extend from the skin to the facial skeleton, or false, which connect only the muscles to the bone and do not extend superficially to the skin.

HOW TO IDENTIFY THE FACIAL VASCULATURE: THE XYZ CONCEPT OF FACIAL VESSELS

Injectors fear facial vessels and of course want to avoid the injection of filler material into the vascular lumen. Knowledge of anatomy of facial vessels is thus important for any injector.

Most textbooks identify the relative location of each facial vessel in a two-dimensional conceptual manner. The vessel position is an approximation of its course in 2 dimensions on the skin surface (**Fig. 1**). This surface concept can be thought of as locating the vessel on an X–Y grid. However, it is clear to any anatomist that the course of each facial vessel varies in relation to the skin surface. For example, the course of the supraorbital vascular bundle can be approximated as it emerges from the foramen at the supraorbital rim and travels superiorly toward the vertex of the scalp. But, if the left and the right supraorbital vessels courses are compared, they are clearly different. In other words, the X–Y location of the vessel is variant. The nonconsistent location of each vessel in relation to the skin surface causes every injector to worry (see **Fig. 1**).

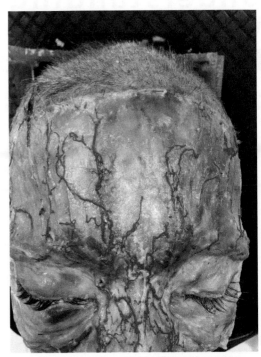

Fig. 1. Upper facial dissection of a latex injected body donor: This demonstrates the supratrochlear and supraorbital arteries coursing vertically over the frontalis. It is clear that the depth or Z plane of the arteries is the same bilaterally, but the vessels in the X–Y plane are not symmetric between the left and right sides of the face.

However, the depth of each facial vessel is consistent and predictable. The vessel depth can be thought of as the Z plane. Injectors can use this knowledge of the vessel depth (Z plane) to identify the vessel course and avoid intravascular injection. A perfect example of this is the course of the supraorbital and supratrochlear vessels. The vessels exit the supraorbital foramen or notch at the medial aspect of the superior orbital rim and travel superiorly to supply the forehead and scalp. The arteries give off several small branches as they course through the forehead and scalp. However, the course of each supraorbital or supratrochlear artery is variable. This is evidenced by noticing the significant difference between the course of the arteries in the left versus the right side of any individual. Thus, the course in the X–Y plane is variable and unpredictable. The variability in course of arteries in the X–Y plane is daunting and scary to all injectors.

The depth of the arteries, however, is very predictable. The supraorbital and supratrochlear arteries are deep (at the level of the bone) at the supraorbital rim. As the arteries travel superiorly, they become more superficial. Specifically, the arteries exit the canal or foramen and quickly pierce the body of the corrugator supercilius muscle. The arteries then pierce the frontalis muscle and travel superiorly on the superficial surface of the frontalis muscle. This course and transition from deep to superficial is very consistent and predictable and allows the injector to avoid the vessel by injecting filler either superficial or deep to vessel.

The same concept can be applied to the facial artery. The facial artery begins deep in the neck giving off several branches and becomes more superficial by piercing the platysma. Then it can be found crossing the body of the mandible anterior to the masseter muscle, which is relatively superficial compared with its origin, but deep in relation to its course on the face. At the point that the artery crosses the mandible, it is deep on bone, deep to the platysma. At this location, it is typically possible to palpate the artery as well as the anterior border of the masseter. Once the facial artery gives off branches in the face, these branches are variable in their X–Y plane, but again predictable in the Z plane. For example, the inferior labial artery is deep to the depressor anguli oris muscle and pierces through the orbicularis oris muscle making it more superficial.[1] The artery particularly becomes superficial near the nose at the angular artery and lateral nasal artery, but it becomes deeper in the lip. The injector can be aware of the Z plane of the vessels at these locations to guide safe injecting by again being either deep or superficial to the vessel. Injecting in the midface is typically performed deeper which avoids injection in or near these vessels (**Fig. 2**).

In another example, the concept of the Z plane can be applied to the superficial temporal artery, especially when injecting in the temple. The depth (Z plane) of the main trunk of the artery is consistently layer III. In regards to the temple, an injector can safely avoid vascular compromise with the injection of filler primarily by going deeper than this plane and occasionally much more superficial. Although there will be variation in the artery and its branches in the X–Y plane, the Z plane is predictable and allows for safe injecting (**Fig. 3**).

PERTINENT VASCULATURE
External carotid artery branches

Facial artery
The facial artery is one of the most important arteries supplying the facial tissues. It is a branch of the external carotid artery and supplies much of the superficial face after providing supply to the neck. After coursing over the mandible and just anterior to the masseter the facial artery has a tortuous course and gives off the superior and inferior labial arteries, the lateral nasal artery, and the angular artery which is typically a terminal branch.[2] Given known variation in the termination of the artery, groupings have been developed based on the artery which is the terminal branch to designate different types of the artery.[3] These branches supply a large portion of the midface including the nose, lips, and cheeks. The facial artery and its branches have a close relationship with the facial musculature and the superficial musculoaponeurotic system (SMAS). It is typically deep to the zygomaticus major and risorius, superficial to the buccinator and levator anguli oris, and may pierce the levator labii superioris until it reaches its termination in the levator labii superioris alaeque.

There is significant anastomosis between bilateral facial arteries as well as with the internal carotid artery branches. There is also variation in anatomy between patients and between each side of the face. For example, in some circumstances, the angular artery is not the terminal branch and may originate from the ophthalmic artery instead.[4] The relationship of the facial artery to the layers of the face as well as the knowledge that of the anastomosis with the

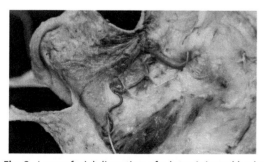

Fig. 2. Lower facial dissection of a latex injected body donor exposing the left facial side: This cadaveric dissection demonstrates the facial artery as it crosses deep on bone anterior to the masseter and then becomes more superficial in the face.

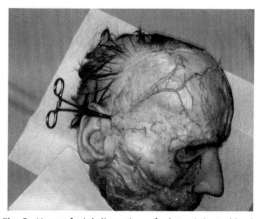

Fig. 3. Upper facial dissection of a latex injected body donor exposing the right temple: Superficial Temporal Artery in layer III on a cadaveric dissection with the skin and subcutaneous tissue (layers I and II) removed.

internal carotid artery and the ophthalmic artery branch is helpful for avoiding vascular compromise with injections in the midface.[5]

Although there is collateral circulation between sides of the face, one area that may be more subject to vascular compromise due to compression or intra-arterial injection is the nasal tip or ala due to more limited collateral circulation for the alar branch of the angular arteries.[6]

Again, using the XYZ plane concept, an injector can avoid this complication with knowledge of the consistent Z plane of the artery at the sites of injection. The artery is consistently deep over as it crosses the mandible, more superficial in the midface, and nose and deeper in the lip.

Superficial temporal artery

The superficial temporal artery is a terminal branch of the external carotid artery. This is an artery that many injectors may not consider to be as important or dangerous to avoid when injecting filler. It is frequently encountered during rhytidectomy. It courses from near the external auditory canal and parotid gland anteriorly and superiorly over the zygoma, then dividing into frontal and parietal branches. It travels within layer III, which is primarily the temporoparietal fascia at the main trunk of this artery. There is an anastomosis between the superficial temporal artery frontal branch and the supraorbital and supratrochlear arteries which explains how devastating consequences can result from injection into this artery.[7] (see **Fig. 3**; **Fig. 4**)

Internal carotid artery branches

Supratrochlear and supraorbital arteries

The supratrochlear and supraorbital arteries are branches of the internal carotid artery that provide

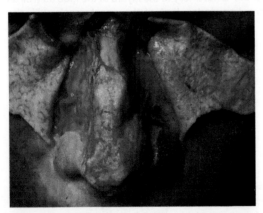

Fig. 4. Nasal dissection of a latex injected body donor: This is a cadaveric example of the nasal vascular anatomy with the skin and subcutaneous tissue removed. This demonstrates how the vessels between each side are significantly different in their course and orientation, but that they are at the same depth.

vascular supply to the face. As described above, they have a consistent origin and depth (Z plane), but can have variability in the XY plane.

Supratrochlear artery

A terminal branch of the ophthalmic artery, the supratrochlear artery, exits at the medial supraorbital rim either through a foramen or a notch and travels vertically over the forehead. It pierces the orbital septum 1.7 to 2.2 cm from the midline giving branching into superficial and deep branches proximal to the corrugator supercilii. The superficial branch becomes superficial to the frontalis muscle and the galea to the subcutaneous plane, while the deep branch can be found in a subgaleal plane if it exists as there can be variation between people.[8]

Supraorbital artery

The supraorbital artery is also a branch of the ophthalmic artery which exits through the supraorbital foramen and divides into 2 terminal branches, superficial and deep. It typically is located about 2 to 3.2 cm from the midline on either side as it crosses the orbital rim.[9] This artery also anastomoses with the contralateral system as well as the supratrochlear and superficial temporal arteries.[10–13]

As discussed in the previous section, both arteries may vary in their XY plane; however, they are predictable in the Z plane which makes it possible to inject safely without arterial compromise which could lead to devastating effects.

Techniques for safe injecting

The knowledge of possible vascular complications related to injections can be intimidating, but the knowledge of the vascular anatomy and the layers of the face can prevent such a devastating complication. Understanding the arteries in relation to the layers of the face and their location in the Z plane provides extremely helpful information to the injector about how to avoid vascular compromise in any area of the face. The injector can use this information to perform injections either deep or superficial to this Z plane for which the artery resides.

SUMMARY

Facial rejuvenation with injectable fillers is common and increasing in demand and use. There are risks to the use of injectable fillers which unfortunately include vascular compromise due to intraluminal injection or compression. Avoiding intraluminal injection is paramount to any injector. Using the applied anatomy of the vasculature of the face, the injector is able to succeed with this.

The anatomy of the vasculature of the face can be topographically difficult to predict. However, the depth of the vessels is well established and very predictable. In this article, we have provided several anatomic examples and their practical correlates for understanding and applying an understanding of the vasculature of the face for safe injecting.

CLINICS CARE POINTS

- There are risks to the use of injectable fillers which unfortunately include vascular compromise due to intraluminal injection or compression.

- The anatomy of the vasculature of the face can be topographically difficult to predict.

- Thorough knowledge of the layered anatomy allows the practitioner to apply techniques that avoid intravascular injection and their associated vascular complications.

DISCLOSURES

The authors have nothing to disclose.

REFERENCES

1. Shahid S. Facial artery. Kenhub GmbH; 2021. Available at: https://www.kenhub.com/en/library/anatomy/facial-artery. Accessed January 10, 2022.

2. Meegalla N, Sood G, Nessel TA, et al. Anatomy, Head and neck, facial arteries. In: StatPearls. Treasure Island (FL): StatPearls Publishing; 2022.

3. Pavithran R. Cadaveric study of branches of facial artery in the face. Int J Curr Res Rev 2022. https://doi.org/10.31782/IJCRR.2021.14107.

4. Koziej M, Trybus M, Holda M, et al. Anatomical map of the facial artery for facial reconstruction and aesthetic procedures. Aesthet Surg J 2019;39(11):1151–62.

5. Standring S. The anatomy of the vascular and lymphatic systems. In: Gray's anatomy the anatomical basis of clinical practice. 42nd edition. London: Elsevier Limited; 2021. p. 1464.e6-9.

6. Injectable fillers of the face. In: Papel I, Frodel J, Holt R, et al, editors. Facial plastic and reconstructive surgery. 4th edition. New York: Thieme; 2016.

7. Hou K, Guo Y, Xu K, et al. Clinical importance of the superficial temporal artery in neurovascular diseases: A PRISMA-compliant systematic review. Int J Med Sci 2019;16(10):1377–85.

8. Agorgianitis L, Panagouli E, Tsakotos G, et al. The Supratrochlear artery revisited: an anatomic review in favor of modern cosmetic applications in the area. Cureus 2020;12(2):e7141.

9. Erdogmus S, Govsa F. Anatomy of the supraorbital region and the evaluation of it for the reconstruction of facial defects. J Craniofac Surg 2007;18(1):104–12.

10. Gruijicic R. Supraorbital artery. Kenhub GmbH. 2021. Available at: https://www.kenhub.com/en/library/anatomy/supraorbital-artery. Accessed January 10, 2022.

11. Sykes JM. Applied anatomy of the temporal region and forehead for injectable fillers. J Drugs Dermatol 2009;8(10 suppl):s24–7.

12. Sykes JM, Cotofana S, Trevidic P, et al. Upper face: clinical anatomy and regional approaches with injectable fillers. Plast Reconstr Surg 2015;136(5 suppl):204S–18S.

13. Sykes JM, Allak A, Palhazi P, et al. Anatomy for facial fillers: the skin surface and beyond. Basel: Dermal Fillers; 2018.

Virtual Surgical Planning (VSP) in Craniomaxillofacial Reconstruction

Krishna Vyas, MD, PhD, MHS[a], Waleed Gibreel, MBBS[a], Samir Mardini, MD[b],*

KEYWORDS

- Virtual surgical planning • Facial reconstruction • Craniomaxillofacial surgery • Craniofacial surgery
- 3D printing • Orthognathic surgery • Cranial vault remodeling • Craniosynostosis

KEY POINTS

- The restoration of the complex three-dimensional (3D) anatomy of the craniomaxillofacial skeleton creates a unique challenge for the reconstructive surgeon.
- The advent of virtual surgical planning (VSP) through computer-aided design (CAD) and computer-aided manufacturing (CAM) has advanced reconstructive outcomes in craniomaxillofacial aesthetic and reconstructive surgery.
- VSP has allowed for precise preoperative planning and decreased the necessity for intraoperative trial and error, often resulting in reduced operating room time and improved outcomes compared to traditional techniques.
- Planning through virtual surgery, 3D printing of stereolithographic models, manufacturing of cutting guides, prefabricated reconstruction plates, and refinements of custom implants help facilitate the execution of spatially complex reconstructions such as craniosynostosis, cranial vault remodeling (CVR), maxillary and mandibular reconstruction, and orthognathic surgery.

INTRODUCTION

Craniomaxillofacial reconstruction poses unique challenges due to the 3D configuration and the importance to restore function (speech, mastication, swallowing, breathing, facial animation) and aesthetics. Virtual Surgical Planning (VSP) coupled with computer-aided design (CAD) and computer-aided modeling (CAM) have had a major impact in craniomaxillofacial surgery.[1–7] Although the technology has been present for decades for various indications from trauma to oncologic reconstruction, recent advancements have made it more relevant to craniomaxillofacial surgery. Improvement in the resolution and quality of data derived from computed tomography (CT) or magnetic

resonance imaging (MRI) scans have enhanced the virtual environment and creation of three-dimensional (3D) models for surgical planning and manipulation. Surgeons can use models preoperatively to visualize, analyze, and manipulate spatial relationships in multiple dimensions and to trial different surgical approaches such as determining the placement of osteotomies and bone grafts, thereby increasing accuracy, efficiency and reducing operative time. Improved outcomes of actual versus planned volume changes, osseous overlap, and aesthetics have been reported.[8] 3D models can be augmented with soft tissue structures (such as nerves and blood vessels) to further plan for complex cases. VSP and 3D printing of surgical models and guides may

[a] Division of Plastic Surgery, Department of Surgery, Mayo Clinic, Rochester, MN, USA; [b] Division of Plastic Surgery, Department of Surgery, Obaid Center for Reconstructive Transplant Surgery, Mayo Clinic, MA1244W, 200 First Street Southwest, Rochester, MN 55905, USA
* Corresponding author. Division of Plastic Surgery, Department of Surgery Surgical Director, Obaid Center for Reconstructive Transplant Surgery, Mayo Clinic, MA1244W, 200 First Street Southwest, Rochester, MN 55905.
E-mail address: Mardini.Samir@mayo.edu

Facial Plast Surg Clin N Am 30 (2022) 239–253
https://doi.org/10.1016/j.fsc.2022.01.016
1064-7406/22/© 2022 Elsevier Inc. All rights reserved.

Box 1
VSP Workflow

Data acquisition from preoperative imaging

Data transfer

Meetings between surgeon and biomedical engineer

Creation of the virtual surgical plan

Design of patient-specific 3D models, guides, and templates

Printing of 3D guides (shipped vs in-house)

Quality control, inspection and delivery

Execution of surgery

help to improve the accuracy and predictability of outcomes in these settings.

VIRTUAL SURGICAL PLANNING AND THREE-DIMENSIONAL-GUIDE CREATION WORKFLOW

In VSP and 3D-printed guides and models creation, a close relationship between the surgeon and biomedical engineers is crucial to yield successful outcomes. One or more meetings are held between the surgeon and engineers to plan the surgery and finalize the design of the 3D-printed guides (**Box 1**). Team communication is critical and checklists may minimize errors in planning. For example, in orthognathic procedures, a typical conversation would include assessment of cephalometrics and osteotomy guides, accuracy of occlusion, midline, facial height, condyle position, and bony contact. Clinical judgment will ultimately guide the virtual plan.

High-resolution CT imaging is the gold standard imaging modality and it serves as a starting point of VSP and 3D printed guide creation. At our institution, sub-millimeter thickness CT scanning is the most commonly used imaging modality for surgical planning. Our group has also studied the accuracy of black bone MRI in the planning and execution of cranial vault remodeling (CVR), orbital floor reconstruction using custom-made plates, and mandibular reconstruction using fibular bone. Blackbone MRI reduces the risks related to radiation exposure and was found to have comparable pragmatic functionality when compared with CT for VSP.[9–15] We are currently evaluating and implementing the clinical use of black bone MRI in VSP and fabrication of 3D models and guides.

The imaging data is sent digitally to a medical modeling facility and then segmented, a process in which borders of anatomic regions in the scan are defined from 2D greyscale images to create a 3D virtual reconstruction. The segmented file is then transferred to a CAD program to assess the accuracy of the 3D images to the axial images. The 3D file is then sent to a biomedical engineer and a VSP session takes place. In craniofacial trauma, a virtual reduction of fractures to normalized anatomy is performed by moving fragments to anatomic configuration in three planes using standard anatomic landmarks, age-matched normative comparisons, or mirror imaging to the contralateral side (if normal). At this stage, numerical values such as anatomic distances, bone thickness, intracranial volumes, and orbital volume can be assessed to aid with pertinent surgical steps such as osteotomies and hardware fixation. The VSP is put through slicing software so the 3D model can be manufactured by a 3D printer. Non-sterilizable 3D models can be used for pre-operative education and use printer technologies such as binder jetting, material jetting, and sheet lamination. If sterilizable 3D models are required for intraoperative use, powder bed fusion and vat polymerization are used. At our institution, for example, an in-house sterilizable 3DP model can be made using vat photopolymerization on a Form3B Form Labs stereolithography 3D printer (Formlabs, Boston, MA) using Formlabs Surgical Resin, which is biocompatible and autoclave sterilizable. The model is then processed (through processes such as alcohol washes, lye baths, water jets, or photocuring), evaluated for quality control, and provided to the surgeon.

CRANIOSYNOSTOSIS

The goals of CVR in craniosynostosis are to increase intracranial volume to allow for continued brain growth, to reduce or prevent increased intracranial pressure, and to restore a normal cranial vault morphology. CVR requires the creation of multiple osteotomies and intraoperative modifications of the position of bone segments to create an expanded cranial vault that has a normal morphology. The phenotype of each craniosynostosis is different and subtle differences do exist even among patients with the same fused suture.[16–18] Modifications and variations of the surgical technique are necessary to account for these morphologic variations. CAD–CAM technology for craniosynostosis was first proposed in 1996, and multiple evolutions and applications ensued over time. Age-matched normative calvarial models were developed years later and were directly compared with data obtained from the patient's CT. The normative model and patient model are then overlapped. VSP is used to simulate osteotomies and repositioning of bone segments during

CVR to best match the normative skull morphology. Cutting and positioning guides and templates are then designed and fabricated to reflect whereby osteotomies should be performed on the calvarium, denoting the location of the sagittal sinus (**Fig. 1**).[19] Positioning guides and registration blocks position reconstruction back onto skull base (**Fig. 2**) and allow for the placement of individual bone segments to approximate an age-appropriate normative calvarial morphology.[20]

VSP also allows the surgeon to acquire quantitative values regarding the anticipated changes in cranial dimensions including the increase in intracranial volume following vault expansion. Analysis of the virtually planned postoperative skull allows us to anticipate bone gaps and to plan appropriately. The spatial relation of the new construct to the skull base is an essential consideration. Integrated reference points in the VSP and cutting/positioning guides allow for the alignment of these points when placing the new construct into the final position and before external plating and fixation.[5]

VSP allows for the surgeon to rehearse the operative plan which helps to anticipate potential problems. In other words, the surgeon knows the outcome before executing the surgical procedure. The virtual surgical plan is used to educate the patient and family through virtual images and 3D models. Furthermore, plate bending and fixation

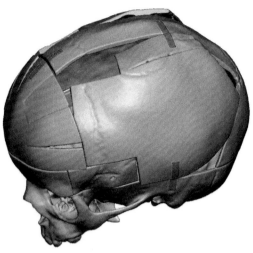

Fig. 2. Positioning guides and registration blocks position reconstruction back onto skull base. (*Courtesy of* Krishna Vyas, MD, PhD, MHS, Minnesota, Waleed Gibreel, MBBS, Minnesota and Samir Mardini, MD, Minnesota)

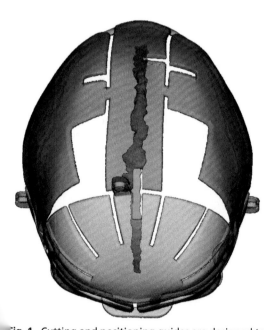

Fig. 1. Cutting and positioning guides are designed to reflect whereby osteotomies should be performed on the calvarium, denoting the location of the sagittal sinus. (*Courtesy of* Krishna Vyas, MD, PhD, MHS, Minnesota, Waleed Gibreel, MBBS, Minnesota and Samir Mardini, MD, Minnesota)

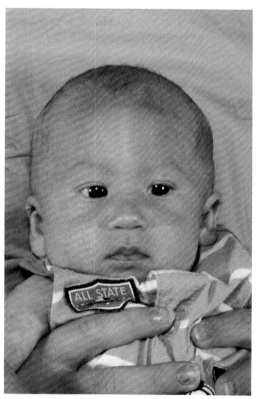

Fig. 3. Preoperative photographs of a 2-month-old male with metopic synostosis. (*Courtesy of* Krishna Vyas, MD, PhD, MHS, Minnesota, Waleed Gibreel, MBBS, Minnesota and Samir Mardini, MD, Minnesota)

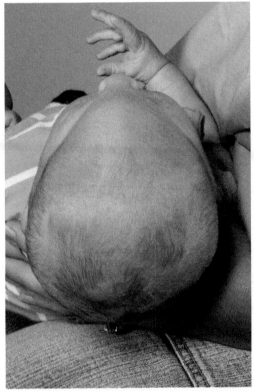

Fig. 4. Preoperative photographs of a 2-month-old male with metopic synostosis.

can be taught to surgical trainees outside of the operating room, thereby saving time under anesthesia for the patient and cost.

Preoperative photographs of a 2-month-old male with a metopic synostosis are shown. (**Figs. 3–5**). 3D modeling and VSP are performed and a 3D printed template is created (**Fig. 6**) with proposed osteotomies (**Fig. 7**). The cutting guides help with positioning of osteotomies on the calvarium (**Fig. 8,9**). The positioning guides, which are based on age- and gender-appropriate

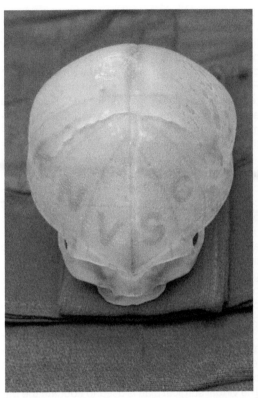

Fig. 6. 3D printed skull derived from 3D reconstructed CT and simulated VSP showing the preoperative anatomy. (*Courtesy of* Krishna Vyas, MD, PhD, MHS, Minnesota, Waleed Gibreel, MBBS, Minnesota and Samir Mardini, MD, Minnesota)

normative measurements, guide the placement of individual bone pieces to achieve a normal calvarial morphology. The bone segments are placed on the inside of the guides and secured with resorbable plates (**Figs. 10 and 11**). The reconstructed calvarium is then transferred to the patient and secured further with resorbable plates

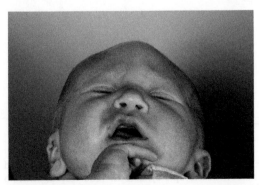

Fig. 5. Preoperative photographs of a 2-month-old male with metopic synostosis.

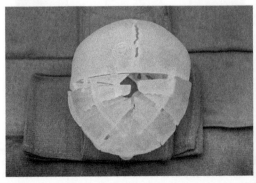

Fig. 7. 3D printed skull showing the postoperative anatomy. (*Courtesy of* Krishna Vyas, MD, PhD, MHS, Minnesota, Waleed Gibreel, MBBS, Minnesota and Samir Mardini, MD, Minnesota)

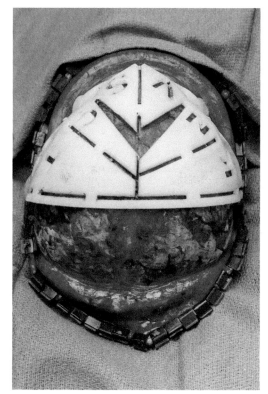

Fig. 8. The cutting guides allow precise placement of osteotomies and labeling of individual bone segments in a patient with metopic synostosis. Placement of the guide on the calvarium after the incision and elevation of the scalp flaps. (*Courtesy of* Krishna Vyas, MD, PhD, MHS, Minnesota, Waleed Gibreel, MBBS, Minnesota and Samir Mardini, MD, Minnesota)

to provide rigid support (**Fig. 12**). Premolding of resorbable plates can be performed on a model to decrease operative time. One month (**Figs. 13–15**) and 7-year (**Figs. 16–18**) postoperative photographs are shown.

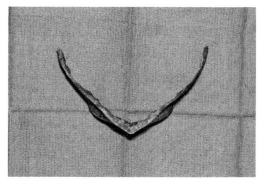

Fig. 9. The supraorbital bandeau showing the triangulation of the forehead. (*Courtesy of* Krishna Vyas, MD, PhD, MHS, Minnesota, Waleed Gibreel, MBBS, Minnesota and Samir Mardini, MD, Minnesota)

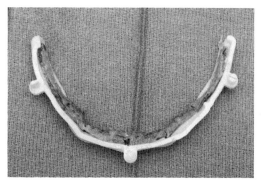

Fig. 10. The remodelled bandeau isplaced on the internal surface of the positioning guide and secured with resorbable plates. (*Courtesy of* Krishna Vyas, MD, PhD, MHS, Minnesota, Waleed Gibreel, MBBS, Minnesota and Samir Mardini, MD, Minnesota)

CRANIAL VAULT DISTRACTION

Posterior cranial vault distraction is a frequently performed surgery in multiple-suture synostosis often present in syndromic patients. This procedure can be performed either before or after anterior CVR with the goal of increasing the intracranial volume to reduce elevated intracranial pressure. VSP helps to guide distractor placement, vectors, and distance of distraction, thereby permitting maximum expansion while guiding the location of osteotomies and optimizing the final shape. VSP provides numeric values of the preoperative and postoperative intracranial volumes which help with the estimation of the predicted increase in intracranial volume. The increase in the intracranial volume is directly proportional to the distraction distance. Therefore, the decision regarding total distraction distance can be guided by objective data related to the anticipated increase in intracranial volume. Calvarial bone thickness can also be calculated virtually to determine the length of screws to be used.

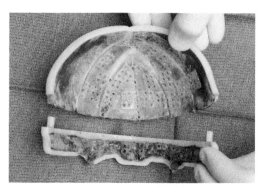

Fig. 11. Bone segments are placed on the internal surface of the positioning guide and secured with resorbable plates.

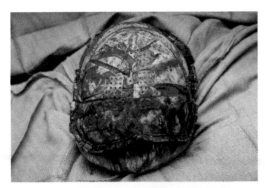

Fig. 12. The reconstructed calvarium is transferred to the patient and further secured with resorbable plates on the external aspect. (*Courtesy of* Krishna Vyas, MD, PhD, MHS, Minnesota, Waleed Gibreel, MBBS, Minnesota and Samir Mardini, MD, Minnesota)

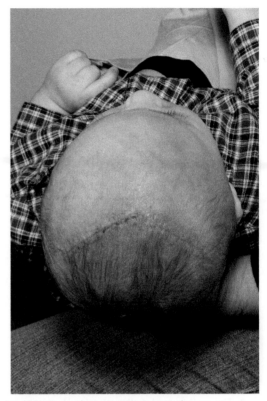

Fig. 14. 1-month postoperative results.

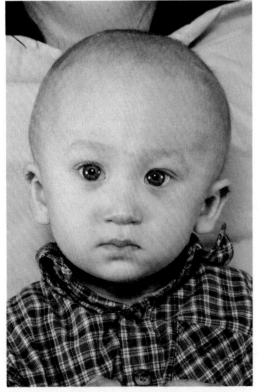

Fig. 13. 1-month postoperative results. (*Courtesy of* Krishna Vyas, MD, PhD, MHS, Minnesota, Waleed Gibreel, MBBS, Minnesota and Samir Mardini, MD, Minnesota)

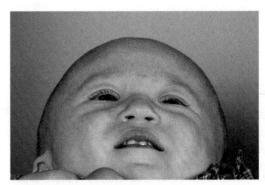

Fig. 15. 1-month postoperative results.

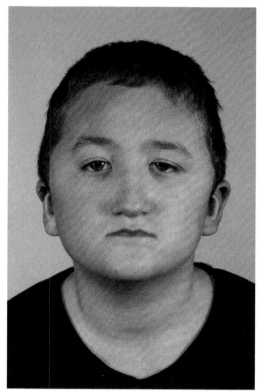

Fig. 16. 7-year postoperative results. (*Courtesy of* Krishna Vyas, MD, PhD, MHS, Minnesota, Waleed Gibreel, MBBS, Minnesota and Samir Mardini, MD, Minnesota)

Chiari malformation is frequently seen in patients with syndromic, multiple-suture craniosynostosis. When posterior vault distraction is performed in these patients, a very low osteotomy (below the transverse venous sinus) allows for posterior fossa volume expansion which can improve the Chiari malformation. With the use of VSP and 3D models, the transverse venous sinus can be clearly visualized and low osteotomy can be placed below the sinus to avoid sinus injury.[21,22] VSP is also used for frontofacial distraction and midface distraction to guide the location of osteotomies and vector of distraction.

MANDIBULAR DISTRACTION

VSP has been used in planning mandibular distraction osteogenesis in neonates with Pierre Robin sequence.[22] Three-D models fabricated from imaging data of the craniofacial skeleton allow for accurate planning of mandibular osteotomies and the distraction vector. Cutting guides are then fabricated to allow for accurate osteotomies away from the inferior alveolar nerve and dental roots. The guides can allow sliding of the

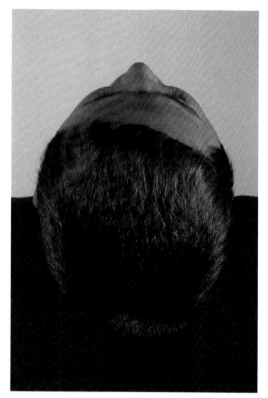

Fig. 17. 7-year postoperative results.

distractors over K-wires to improve the accuracy of placement of the distractors. Screws position and lenght can be planned to ensure bicortical placement away from the inferior alveolar nerve and developing dental follicles.

COMPLEX MAXILLOFACIAL RECONSTRUCTION

Advances in imaging and VSP over the past decade have allowed high-fidelity reproduction of complex malformations and tumors and adjacent structures involved in the resection and

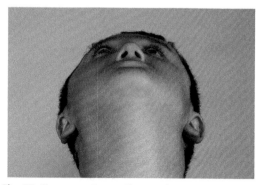

Fig. 18. 7-year postoperative results.

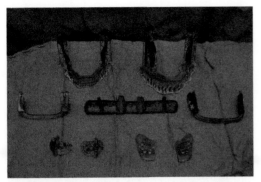

Fig. 19. With imaging data from high-resolution CT scans of the maxillofacial skeleton and lower extremity, 3D models are created. (*Courtesy of* Krishna Vyas, MD, PhD, MHS, Minnesota, Waleed Gibreel, MBBS, Minnesota and Samir Mardini, MD, Minnesota)

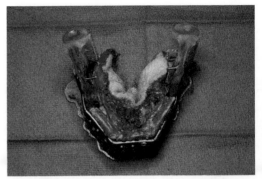

Fig. 21. Plate-bending template for shaping the fibula to the reconstructed mandible. (*Courtesy of* Krishna Vyas, MD, PhD, MHS, Minnesota, Waleed Gibreel, MBBS, Minnesota and Samir Mardini, MD, Minnesota)

reconstruction. High-resolution imaging and CAD–CAM software allow the reproduction of 3D models of the tumor with pertinent anatomic structures and vasculature, facilitating multidisciplinary discussion among ablative and reconstructive surgeons and patients.[23] As "in-house" 3D printing technologies become more accessible and time-efficient indications may expand to more acute trauma settings. Challenges with in-house production do exist, however, as anatomic modeling and printing units require a dedicated and compliant space with quality control measures, infrastructure, and training of personnel.

In a study comparing midface defects reconstructed with subscapular system free flaps with VSP and without VSP, VSP was found to be associated with improved subunit reconstruction, bony segment contact, and anatomically correct bone segment positioning.[24]

In multiple meta-analyses, VSP and CAD/CAM has been found to decrease operating room

time and ischemia time with no difference in complications such as nonunion, flap loss, microvascular complications, or hardware-related complications.[25,26]

MAXILLARY AND MANDIBULAR RECONSTRUCTION

VSP and CAD/CAM offer many benefits in oncologic head and neck reconstruction. Traditionally, reconstructive outcomes relied on surgical experience, skill, and intraoperative trial-and-error to create a neomandible or neomaxilla. Preoperative communication between the ablative and reconstructive team was often limited by discussion of the precise anatomy of the resection site, which became apparent only in the operating room.

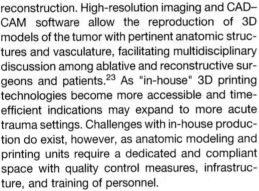

Fig. 20. Mandibular and fibular cutting guides. (*Courtesy of* Krishna Vyas, MD, PhD, MHS, Minnesota, Waleed Gibreel, MBBS, Minnesota and Samir Mardini, MD, Minnesota)

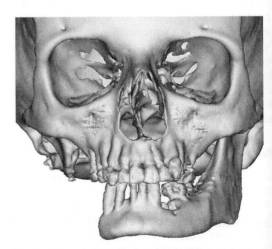

Fig. 22. Frontal view of preoperative anatomy. (*Courtesy of* Krishna Vyas, MD, PhD, MHS, Minnesota, Waleed Gibreel, MBBS, Minnesota and Samir Mardini, MD, Minnesota)

VSP CAD/CAM has been shown to enhance communication among surgical teams and patients, thereby progressing confidently with a definitive surgical plan.

In the area of mandibular reconstruction, VSP has been used in the shaping of free vascularized bone flaps.[27,28] With imaging data from high-resolution CT scans of the maxillofacial skeleton and lower extremity, 3D models can be crafted (**Fig. 19**) and virtual surgery can allow for the fabrication of mandibular and fibular cutting guides (**Fig. 20**) and a plate-bending template for the shaping of the fibula to the reconstructed mandible (**Fig. 21**).

With VSP, intraoperative and flap ischemia time can be decreased with preoperative planning of fibular osteotomies and preoperative hardware bending and manipulation.[29] When immediate dental implants are placed, the location and number of implants can be determined preoperatively. Placement guides allow the precise placement of these implants. Osteotomies, bone fixation, and implant placement can all be performed in situ while the flap is still perfused which minimizes ischemia time. The accuracy of these fibular osteotomies and implant placement optimizes positioning for future dental rehabilitation.

A case of right hemimandibulectomy to treat osteoradionecrosis following radiation treatment of tonsillar carcinoma is demonstrated. High-resolution CT scans of the maxillofacial skeleton are used to generate a 3D reconstruction (**Figs. 22 and 23**). A left free fibula graft to the right mandible with intraoral skin paddle is planned using VSP. The VSP for mandibular cutting guides with metal slot inserts and predictive holes (**Figs.**

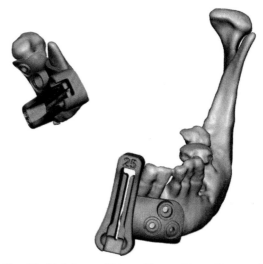

Fig. 24. Metal mandible cutting guides with metal slot inserts and predictive holes. (*Courtesy of* Krishna Vyas, MD, PhD, MHS, Minnesota, Waleed Gibreel, MBBS, Minnesota and Samir Mardini, MD, Minnesota)

24 and 25) and fibular cutting guide with metal slot inserts are shown (**Figs. 26–28**). VSP also simulates the mandibular hardware with predictive holes for positioning (**Fig. 29**). Fibular guides assist with osteotomies (**Fig. 30**) and inset (**Fig. 31**). Proposed postoperative anatomy is also simulated via VSP (**Figs. 32 and 33**).

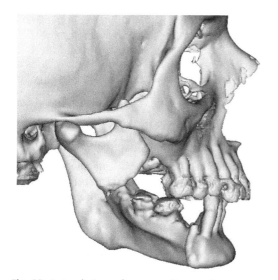

Fig. 23. Lateral view of preoperative anatomy.

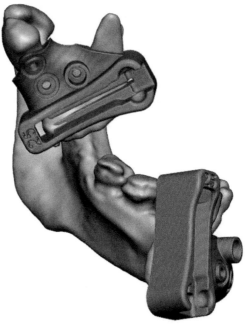

Fig. 25. Metal mandible cutting guides with metal slot inserts and predictive holes.

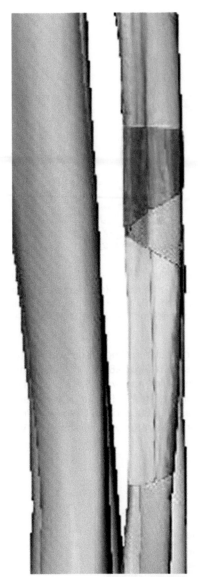

Fig. 26. Sites of fibula osteotomies . (*Courtesy of Krishna Vyas, MD, PhD, MHS, Minnesota, Waleed Gibreel, MBBS, Minnesota and Samir Mardini, MD, Minnesota*)

VSP can be applied to other free vascularized flaps donor sites such as the scapula and iliac crest. In a recent meta-analysis of mandibular reconstruction with free fibular flaps, VSP-guided

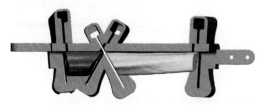

Fig. 27. Fibula cutting guide with metal slot inserts.

reconstructions were associated with significantly decreased operative time (by 44.6 minutes). No statistical difference between cohorts for major or minor complications was identified and there was insufficient data for cost analysis and accuracy due to lack of standardized measurements.[30–32] Another meta-analysis also reported significantly decreased intraoperative time and ischemic time compared with non-VSP cohorts in fibular free flaps for head and neck reconstruction. VSP was also associated with reduced orthognathic deviation from the ideal outcome when compared with conventional techniques. Again, no statistically significant differences in complication rates were identified.[33] These findings are reaffirmed when comparing head and neck reconstructions.

ORTHOGNATHIC SURGERY

VSP and CAD/CAM is a useful technology in orthognathic procedures.[34] Patient-specific virtual and 3D printed models can improve the planning phase. Preoperative simulation of the maxillo-mandibular relationship facilitates the alignment of the proper dental and skeletal relationship. VSP aides with the fabrication of intermediate and final splints to allow the optimal positioning of the maxillary and mandibular segments. In addition, both maxillary and mandibular osteotomies can be executed with the guidance of cutting guides. Custom-made, prebent plates can be fabricated and used for skeletal fixation. Premade guides for autografts and customized hardware such as prebent plates can further promote accurate and predictable translational movements in the operating room. In a systematic review of VSP in orthognathic surgery evaluating nearly 400 articles in the literature, accuracy analyses had an average translation (<2 mm) in the maxilla and in the mandible (in 3 planes[35]). The accuracy values for pitch, yaw, and roll (°) were (<2.75, < 1.7 and < 1.1) for the maxilla and (<2.75, < 1.8, < 1.1) for the mandible, respectively. When comparing VSP with traditional planning, VSP was more accurate, specifically for frontal symmetry. VSP and 3D surgical splints facilitate diagnosis, treatment planning and accuracy, dentofacial deformity class, planning vectors, advancement distances, occlusal splints, surgical techniques, type of advancement, or asymmetry.[36]

Cutting and positioning guides can also be used to plan and execute osseous genioplasty. Cutting guides permit the execution of an osteotomy that is below the mental nerve and dental roots and above the genial tuberosity. Prebent plates used for fixation enhance the accuracy of genioplasty.

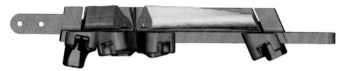

Fig. 28. Fibula cutting guide with metal slot inserts.

CRANIOMAXILLOFACIAL TRAUMA

VSP CAD/CAM has been used for the reconstruction of traumatic craniomaxillofacial injuries ranging from enophthalmos correction in orbital floor fractures to panfacial fracture repair. Panfacial fractures present a special challenge as the spatial relationship between the mandible and maxilla is disrupted. VSP and 3D modeling facilitate the restoration of this relationship via fabrication of intermediate and final dental splints that allow consecutive fixation of the maxilla and mandible. If the patient has a pretrauma CT scan of the maxillofacial skeleton, that scan can be used as a reference to re-establish the premorbid dental and skeletal relationship. When VSP is used for the restoration of the dental and maxillary/mandibular skeletal relationship, additional information about the maxillary and mandibular dentition is needed. In the trauma setting, it is difficult to obtain maxillary and mandibular impressions for different reasons. In these cases, a cone beam CT scan (CBCT) or intraoral digital scanners can be a helpful substitute. Prebent fixation plates decrease intraoperative trial-and-error and often improve operative time. Furthermore, it limits the extent of subperiosteal dissection, minimizing vascularization of bony fragments.

The use of VSP in orbital reconstruction deserves special mention. Enophthalmos following orbital fractures can occur due to an increase in intraorbital volume or decrease of the intraorbital fat volume or both. It is important to know which one is contributing to enophthalmos as correcting the bony orbital volume alone may not result in complete enophthalmos correction in patients with severe atrophy of the periorbital fat. CT scan is valuable in evaluating both the bone anatomy as well as the intraorbital soft tissue. Based on the information obtained from imaging, custommade plates can be fabricated to restore the intraorbital bone volume that takes into account the degree of soft tissue atrophy.

VASCULARIZED COMPOSITE ALLOGRAFT (FACE TRANSPLANTATION)

Face transplant recipients often have challenging craniofacial anatomy due to the initial defect as well as prior attempts at reconstruction. VSP can be particularly helpful in preoperative planning for complex craniomaxillofacial reconstructions such as facial transplantation.[37,38] This includes the planning of osteotomies in a controlled environment for which the recipient defect and donor anatomy can be strategically assessed and the operative plan refined. VSP allows for the development of cutting guides and templates are fabricated for the recipient and for the donor. Intraoperative navigation and innovative mixed reality modalities can also aid in surgical decision-making.[39] VSP enables the assessment of challenging recipient anatomy, including the planning of osteotomies to avoid previously placed reconstructive hardware and plates. It also enables the reconstruction of donor–recipient size mismatches, which may allow for a larger pool of acceptable donors for consideration. Donor osteotomy guides enable cuts to be made when the vascular pedicle is intact. Furthermore, cutting guides and positioning guides are reciprocal, which results in more time-efficient, streamlined, and unified intraoperative decision-making, better correlation of the plan between the donor and recipient surgical teams between the donor and recipient surgical teams, and optimal aesthetic and functional outcomes allowing the surgery to be efficient and streamlined.

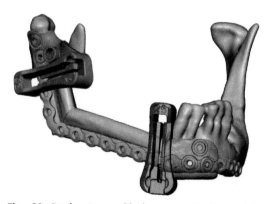

Fig. 29. Pre-bent mandibular reconstruction plate. (*Courtesy of* Krishna Vyas, MD, PhD, MHS, Minnesota, Waleed Gibreel, MBBS, Minnesota and Samir Mardini, MD, Minnesota)

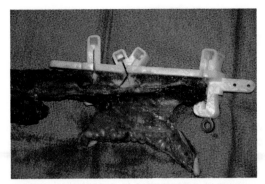

Fig. 30. Cutting guides and completion of fibula osteotomies. (*Courtesy of* Krishna Vyas, MD, PhD, MHS, Minnesota, Waleed Gibreel, MBBS, Minnesota and Samir Mardini, MD, Minnesota)

AESTHETIC SURGERY AND SKELETAL VOLUME AUGMENTATION

VSP can be used to fabricate custom-made implants used for the augmentation of the craniomaxillofacial skeleton such as forehead implants in patients with frontal hypoplasia, zygomatic/midface/pyriform implants in patients with midface and perinasal skeletal and soft tissue deficiency, and mandibular angle and chin implants in patients desiring enhancement in these areas.[40,41]

Facial Feminization Surgery

One of the most significant determinants of gender is the frontonasal–orbital complex, as detailed by Ousterhout from anatomic studies of skulls.[42,43] The male forehead has increased supraorbital bossing, an enlarged frontal sinus, lower and flatter brows, deeper orbits, and a flatter forehead compared with the average female forehead.[44] Preoperative CT and 3D reconstruction before facial feminization surgery helps to delineate

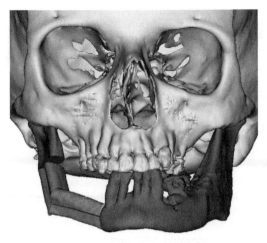

Fig. 32. Frontal view of simulated postoperative anatomy. (*Courtesy of* Krishna Vyas, MD, PhD, MHS, Minnesota, Waleed Gibreel, MBBS, Minnesota and Samir Mardini, MD, Minnesota)

skeletal and sinus anatomy. During preoperative planning, reformatted CT images can be used to generate a 3D printed skeletal model with cutting guides using inexpensive resins. VSP-generated, colored heat maps allow for safe and precise burring or osteotomy with a setback of the frontal bone and allow less intraoperative contouring before repositioning and fixation of the anterior table.[45] VSP allows the surgeon to attempt multiple approaches in a virtual environment, and are invaluable resources during the consultation to educate patients and to review surgical plans.[46] VSP and 3D models aid with the planning and execution of mandibular shaping and genioplasty.

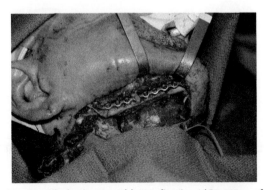

Fig. 31. Fibular inset and bone fixation. (*Courtesy of* Krishna Vyas, MD, PhD, MHS, Minnesota, Waleed Gibreel, MBBS, Minnesota and Samir Mardini, MD, Minnesota)

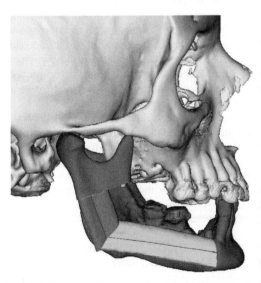

Fig. 33. Lateral view of simulated postoperative anatomy.

SUMMARY

VSP is a technology that holds the potential to predictably advance reconstructive outcomes in craniomaxillofacial aesthetic and reconstructive surgery. This technology can be used for spatially complex surgeries due to its ability to visualize and manipulate 3D configurations of the craniomaxillofacial skeleton. Translational applications continue to expand for cases of varying levels of complexity that require sub-millimeter precision, including orthognathic surgery, oncologic extirpation and reconstruction, congenital differences, aesthetics, and trauma, to improve functional and aesthetic outcomes. Implementation of VSP allows the surgeon to perform preoperative planning and may improve operative predictability, accuracy, precision, efficiency, and reduce operative time. In-house printing of cutting and positioning guides and implants may help reduce the cost and the turn-around time. Advances in software development and 3-D printing will allow for wider applicability. Integration of artificial intelligence could potentially reduce overall time required for production.

Further research regarding cost-effectiveness and long-term aesthetic outcomes are required. Overall, VSP-CAD/CAM has improved accuracy, enabled planning in a less time-sensitive environment, and allowed for effective execution and evaluation of complex reconstructive cases. As more research continues to be performed across surgical disciplines and indications expand, VSP will likely gain more popularity and be adopted by most surgeons performing complex craniomaxillofacial surgeries.

CLINICS CARE POINTS

- Virtual surgical planning combines digital workflows with additive manufacturing and precision surgery to deliver personalized solutions.
- As technology evolves and 3D printing becomes more widely available, refinements and indications may expand to allow for a more accurate and efficient reconstruction of complex craniomaxillofacial deformities.

DISCLOSURE

The authors have nothing to disclose.

REFERENCES

1. Suchyta M, Mardini S. Innovations and Future Directions in Head and Neck Microsurgical Reconstruction. Clin Plast Surg 2017;44(2):325–44.
2. Chim H, Wetjen N, Mardini S. Virtual surgical planning in craniofacial surgery. Semin Plast Surg 2014;28(3):150–8.
3. Sharaf B, Levine J, Hirsch D, et al. Importance of computer-aided design and manufacturing technology in the multidisciplinary approach to head and neck reconstruction. J Craniofac Surg 2010;21(4):1277–80.
4. Pfaff MJ, Steinbacher DM. Plastic surgery applications using three-dimensional planning and computer-assisted design and manufacturing. Plast Reconstr Surg 2016;137(3):603e–16e.
5. Vander Sloten J, Degryse K, Gobin R, et al. Interactive simulation of cranial surgery in a computer aided design environment. J Craniomaxillofac Surg 1996;24(2):122–9.
6. Carlson ER. Virtual Reconstructive Surgical Planning. J Oral Maxillofac Surg 2017;75(1):7–8.
7. Gerstle TL, Ibrahim AM, Kim PS, et al. A plastic surgery application in evolution: three-dimensional printing. Plast Reconstr Surg 2014;133(2):446–51.
8. Rodby K, Turin S, Jacobs R, et al. Advances in Oncologic Head and Neck Reconstruction: Systematic Review and Future Considerations of Virtual Surgical Planning and Computer Aided Design/Computer Aided Modeling. J Plast Reconstr Aesthet Surg 2014;67(9):1171–85.
9. Pearce MS, Salotti JA, Little MP, et al. Radiation exposure from CT scans in childhood and subsequent risk of leukaemia and brain tumours: a retrospective cohort study. Lancet 2012;380(9840):499–505.
10. Domeshek LF, Mukundan S Jr, Yoshizumi T, et al. Increasing concern regarding computed tomography irradiation in craniofacial surgery. Plast Reconstr Surg 2009;123(4):1313–20.
11. Suchyta MA, Gibreel W, Hunt CH, et al. Using Black Bone Magnetic Resonance Imaging in Craniofacial Virtual Surgical Planning: A Comparative Cadaver Study. Plast Reconstr Surg 2018;141(6):1459–70.
12. Eley KA, McIntyre AG, Watt-Smith SR, et al. Black bone" MRI: a partial flip angle technique for radiation reduction in craniofacial imaging. Br J Radiol 2012;85(1011):272–8.
13. Eley KA, Watt-Smith SR, Golding SJ. Black bone" MRI: a potential alternative to CT when imaging the head and neck: report of eight clinical cases and review of the Oxford experience. Br J Radiol 2012;85(1019):1457–64.
14. Eley KA, Watt-Smith SR, Golding SJ. Black Bone" MRI: a potential non-ionizing method for three-dimensional cephalometric analysis–a preliminary

feasibility study. Dentomaxillofac Radiol 2013; 42(10):20130236.

15. Eley KA, Watt-Smith SR, Golding SJ. Black Bone" MRI: a novel imaging technique for 3D printing. Dentomaxillofac Radiol 2017;46(3):20160407.

16. Landes CA, Bitsakis J, Diehl T, et al. Introduction of a three-dimensional anthropometry of the viscerocranium. Part I: measurement of craniofacial development and establishment of standard values and growth functions. J Craniomaxillofac Surg 2002; 30(1):18–24.

17. Landes CA, Zachar R, Diehl T, et al. Introduction of a three-dimensional anthropometry of the viscerocranium. Part II: evaluating osseous and soft tissue changes following orthognathic surgery. J Craniomaxillofac Surg 2002;30(1):25–34.

18. Marcus JR, Domeshek LF, Loyd AM, et al. Use of a three-dimensional, normative database of pediatric craniofacial morphology for modern anthropometric analysis. Plast Reconstr Surg 2009;124(6):2076–84.

19. Khechoyan DY, Saber NR, Burge J, et al. Surgical outcomes in craniosynostosis reconstruction: the use of prefabricated templates in cranial vault re-modelling. J Plast Reconstr Aesthet Surg 2014; 67(1):9–16.

20. Mardini S, Alsubaie S, Cayci C, et al. Three-dimensional preoperative virtual planning and template use for surgical correction of craniosynostosis. J Plast Reconstr Aesthet Surg 2014;67(3):336–43.

21. Iyer RR, Wu A, Macmillan A, et al. Use of computer-assisted design and manufacturing to localize dural venous sinuses during reconstructive surgery for craniosynostosis. Childs Nerv Syst 2018;34(1):137–42.

22. Doscher ME, Garfein ES, Bent J, et al. Neonatal mandibular distraction osteogenesis: converting virtual surgical planning into an operative reality. Int J Pediatr Otorhinolaryngol 2014;78(2):381–4.

23. Bauermeister AJ, Zuriarrain A, Newman MI. Three-Dimensional Printing in Plastic and Reconstructive Surgery: A Systematic Review. Ann Plast Surg 2016;77(5):569–76.

24. Swendseid BP, Roden DF, Vimawala S, et al. Virtual Surgical Planning in Subscapular System Free Flap Reconstruction of Midface Defects. Oral Oncol 2020;101:104508.

25. Padilla PL, Mericli AF, Largo RD, et al. Computer-Aided Design and Manufacturing versus Conventional Surgical Planning for Head and Neck Reconstruction: A Systematic Review and Meta-Analysis. Plast Reconstr Surg 2021;148(1):183–92.

26. Nilsson J, Hindocha N, Thor A. Time matters - Differences between computer-assisted surgery and conventional planning in cranio-maxillofacial surgery: A systematic review and meta-analysis. J Craniomaxillofac Surg 2020;48(2):132–40.

27. Hanasono MM, Skoracki RJ. Computer-assisted design and rapid prototype modeling in microvascular mandible reconstruction. Laryngoscope 2013;123(3):597–604.

28. Antony A, Chen W, Kolokythas A, et al. Use of virtual surgery and stereolithography-guided osteotomy for mandibular reconstruction with the free fibula. Plast Reconstr Surg 2011;128(5):1080–4.

29. Seruya M, Fisher M, Rodriguez E. Computer-Assisted versus Conventional Free Fibula Flap Technique for Craniofacial Reconstruction: An Outcomes Comparison. Plast Reconstr Surg 2013;132(5):1219–28.

30. Glas HH, Vosselman N, de Visscher SAHJ. The use of 3D virtual surgical planning and computer aided design in reconstruction of maxillary surgical defects. Curr Opin Otolaryngol Head Neck Surg 2020;28(2):122–8.

31. Schepers RH, Raghoebar GM, Vissink A, et al. Fully 3-dimensional digitally planned reconstruction of a mandible with a free vascularized fibula and immediate placement of an implant-supported prosthetic construction. Head Neck 2013;35(4):E109–14.

32. Barr ML, Haveles CS, Rezzadeh KS, et al. Virtual Surgical Planning for Mandibular Reconstruction With the Fibula Free Flap: A Systematic Review and Meta-analysis. Ann Plast Surg 2020;84(1):117–22.

33. Tang NSJ, Ahmadi I, Ramakrishnan A. Virtual surgical planning in fibula free flap head and neck reconstruction: A systematic review and meta-analysis. J Plast Reconstr Aesthet Surg 2019;72(9):1465–77.

34. Zinser M, Sailer H, Ritter L, et al. A Paradigm Shift in Orthognathic Surgery? A Comparison of Navigation, Computer-Aided Designed/Computer-Aided Manufactured Splints, and "Classic" Intermaxillary Splints to Surgical Transfer of Virtual Orthognathic Planning. J Oral Maxillofac Surg 2014;72(10):A1–26.

35. Alkhayer A, Piffkó J, Lippold C, et al. Accuracy of virtual planning in orthognathic surgery: a systematic review. Head Face Med 2020;16(1):34.

36. Soncini G, Bolzoni A, Baserga C, et al. Evaluation of factors influencing accuracy of virtual surgical planning in orthognatic surgery. J Biol Regul Homeost Agents 2020;34(5 Suppl. 3).

37. Foley BD, Thayer WP, Honeybrook A, et al. Mandibular Reconstruction Using Computer-Aided Design and Computer-Aided Manufacturing: An Analysis of Surgical Results. J Oral Maxillof Surg 2013;71:e111–9.

38. Chim H, Amer H, Mardini S, et al. Vascularized composite allotransplantation in the realm of regenerative plastic surgery. Mayo Clin Proc 2014;89(7):1009–20.

39. Cho K-H, Papay FA, Yanof J, et al. Mixed Reality and 3D Printed Models for Planning and Execution of Face Transplantation. Ann Surg 2020.

40. Lee JH, Kaban LB, Yaremchuk MJ. Refining Post-Orthognathic Surgery Facial Contour with Computer-Designed/Computer-Manufactured Alloplastic Implants. Plast Reconstr Surg 2018 Sep;142(3):747–55.

41. Straughan DM, Yaremchuk MJ. Changing Mandible Contour Using Computer Designed/Computer Manufactured Alloplastic Implants. Aesthet Surg J 2021 Sep 14;41(10):NP1265–75.
42. Ousterhout DK. Feminization of the forehead: Contour changing to improve female aesthetics. Plast Reconstr Surg 1987;79:701–13.
43. Spiegel JH. Facial determinants of female gender and feminizing forehead cranioplasty. Laryngoscope 2011;121:250–61.
44. Morrison SD, Vyas KS, Motakef S, et al. Facial feminization: Systematic review of the literature. Plast Reconstr Surg 2016;137:1759–70.
45. Sharaf B, Morris J, Vyas KS. Point of Care Virtual Surgical Planning and Three-Dimensional Printing for Feminizing Foreheadplasty. Plast Reconstr Surg 2021;148(6):1080e–2e.
46. Parthasarathy J. 3D modeling, custom implants and its future perspectives in craniofacial surgery. Ann Maxillofac Surg 2014;4:9–18.

Facial Transplantation

Krishna Vyas, MD, PhD, MHS[a], Karim Bakri, MBBS[a], Waleed Gibreel, MBBS[a],
Sebastian Cotofana, MD, PhD[b], Hatem Amer, MD[c,d,e], Samir Mardini, MD[a,d,e],*

KEYWORDS

- Facial transplantation • Vascularized composite allotransplantation • Facial reconstruction
- Craniomaxillofacial surgery • Immunosuppression • Virtual surgical planning • Face transplant
- Microsurgery

KEY POINTS

- Conventional microvascular reconstruction is limited in its capacity to achieve optimal functional and esthetic outcomes when dealing with complex midface neuromotor structures.
- Success in facial transplantation is reliant on patient selection, informed consent, solid psychosocial structure and support, and patient motivation and compliance. A multidisciplinary approach with careful team planning and organization is crucial.
- The decision for face transplantation over conventional reconstructive methods must be considered against the need for lifelong immunosuppression.
- Advances in preoperative planning, virtual surgical planning (VSP), surgical technique, allograft design and refinements, and postoperative revisions have also contributed to optimal results.
- Sharing experiences and outcomes data is essential to accurately estimate complication rates and to compare outcomes.
- Future goals in VCA will include research in tolerance induction and reducing adverse effects associated with immunosuppression.

INTRODUCTION

Facial transplantation is a vascularized composite allotransplantation (VCA) which may be considered in patients with extensive and challenging facial defects for which conventional reconstructive approaches fail to provide satisfactory functional and esthetic outcomes.[1] Historically, options of reconstruction for extensive facial defects, particularly those involving more than one functional unit in the midface, required multiple procedures using techniques such as locoregional flaps and free tissue transfer, and failed to achieve adequate esthetic and functional results. VCA has the advantage of replacing defective or absent structures with anatomically identical tissues. The procedure is both reconstructive and restorative.

The primary goal of facial transplantation is to restore facial form and to improve function. While it is not considered lifesaving, it is considered life-enhancing or life-giving. A face transplant may be considered in patients with severe facial deformities and impaired function of facial structures necessary for facial expression, eating, control of oral secretions, swallowing, speaking, communication, protection of the globe, and other essential functions. As a sensory and expressive organ, the face is an interface with the social world, and most face transplant recipients report improved quality of life and increased social integration.[2]

Facial transplantation can restore multiple structures and tissues, which may include skin, fat, muscles, tendons, cartilage, bones, nerves, blood

[a] Division of Plastic Surgery, Department of Surgery, Mayo Clinic, Rochester, MN, USA; [b] Department of Clinical Anatomy, Mayo Clinic College of Medicine and Science, Mayo Clinic, Rochester, MN, USA; [c] Division of Nephrology and Hypertension, Mayo Clinic, Rochester, MN, USA; [d] Essam and Dalal Obaid Center for Reconstructive Transplant Surgery, Mayo Clinic, Rochester, MN, USA; [e] William J. von Liebig Center for Transplantation and Clinical Regeneration, Mayo Clinic, Rochester, MN, USA
* Corresponding author. Division of Plastic Surgery, Department of Surgery Surgical Director, Obaid Center for Reconstructive Transplant Surgery, Mayo Clinic, MA1244W, 200 First Street Southwest, Rochester, MN 55905.
E-mail address: Mardini.Samir@mayo.edu

Facial Plast Surg Clin N Am 30 (2022) 255–269
https://doi.org/10.1016/j.fsc.2022.01.011

Abbreviations	
VSP	Virtual Surgical Planning
VCA	Vascularized Composite Allotransplantation
3D	Three-Dimensional
CT	Computed Tomography
CAD	Computer-Aided Design
CAM	Computer-Aided Manufacturing
SMAS	Superficial Musculoaponeurotic System

vessels, and mucosa, depending on the reconstructive needs of the recipient. The process of facial transplantation is a long one and requires preparation and commitment on behalf of the patient, caretakers, and other stakeholders.

The first face transplant was performed in Amiens, France in 2005 on a 38-year-old female who sustained severe injuries to the nose, lips, and cheek from a dog bite.[3] The early results were revolutionary and provided hope to patients with facial defects that were considered too severe for reconstruction by conventional procedures. Since then, 48 documented face transplants have been performed worldwide. The most common indications are related to extensive facial trauma, including ballistic injury,[4] burns, and animal attacks.[4–9] Facial transplantation has also been performed to treat benign tumors resulting in significant disfigurement such as neurofibromas.[10–12]

With increased global experience and significant advances in VCA, facial transplantation is increasingly considered as a viable first-line treatment for extensive central facial trauma[13] for which conventional reconstructive options would require multiple procedures and would still fail to provide satisfactory functional and esthetic outcomes.[1,14,15]

OBJECTIVES

This article reviews the following:

- The functional and esthetic importance of the midface.
- Pretransplantation considerations:
  - Multidisciplinary team–based approaches
  - Donor and recipient selection criteria and considerations, including indications and contraindications for facial transplantation
  - Immunologic considerations
  - Ethical considerations
  - Logistical considerations
  - Technical considerations and surgical approaches
- Esthetic, functional, and psychosocial outcomes.
- Lessons learned in facial transplantation.

The Functional and Esthetic Importance of the Midface

Facial transplantation is considered for extensive central avulsive deformities that cannot be repaired adequately through conventional reconstruction methods, such as those with severe composite periorbital, total nasal, or perioral defects. The midface is the foundation for human social, communicative, and emotional function, and is essential to facial identity that is consequently the basis of human relationships. As an organ that expresses emotion, the face represents one's interface with the world. The structures of the face are three-dimensional (3D), unique, and complex. Because the face is composed of a wide range of tissue types, the transfer of autologous tissue to achieve a "normal" look and function is challenging and most of the time impossible, especially in the setting of extensive defects involving unique and delicate structures such as the ocular and oral sphincters, or the vermillion of the lip, which do not have homologs. Even with flap modifications and revisions, there are tremendous limitations to achieving adequate form and function when conventional techniques are performed. Reestablishing the dynamic neuromuscular units of the midface is particularly challenging because free flaps (except for functional muscle transfers such as the gracilis with neurovascular repair) are static structures without natural, purposeful, intrinsic capacity for movement.

PRETRANSPLANTATION CONSIDERATIONS
Multidisciplinary Team–Based Approaches

Facial transplantation epitomizes the concepts of integrative approaches to individualized care.[16] Collaborative multidisciplinary planning is required to rigorously address all aspects of facial transplantation including medical and psychosocial factors. The team consists of facial reconstructive and microsurgeons, transplant physicians, psychiatrists, oculoplastic surgeons, infectious disease specialists, dermatologists, neurologists, rhinologists, anesthesiologists, radiologists, operating room personnel, engineers, dentists, clinical coordinators, social workers, physical therapists, speech therapists, rehabilitation, infectious disease, ophthalmology, clinical anatomists, photographers and videographers, public relation specialists among many other critical members (**Box 1**). Critical to proceeding with a face transplant and every other transplant is a strong collaboration with the regional organ procurement organization (ie, LifeSource).

Donor and Recipient Selection Criteria and Considerations

Facial transplantation is a complex and resource-demanding procedure and proper patient selection is paramount. Several absolute and relative contraindications exist (**Box 2**). The ideal patient will be in good general, physical, and psychological health, and have a solid support system. After initial evaluation with a reconstructive plastic surgeon, a comprehensive and longitudinal psychosocial evaluation is performed by psychiatry and social work. All candidates are evaluated based on motivation, expectations, readiness for life after surgery, compliance, and social support. The recipient must be willing to endure the stresses of the operation and must understand the aggressive postoperative rehabilitation and requirement for lifelong immunosuppression. Psychosocial factors are particularly important for those with self-inflicted injuries or with a history of depression or substance dependence.[17] Mental health should be reassessed continuously to support patient compliance and reduce the risk of allograft failure. A supportive social network is necessary because the process of facial transplantation is long and requires a prolonged postoperative recovery and an intense commitment from patients and caretakers. Strict adherence to a complex medical and rehabilitation regimen is necessary because noncompliance with medications can lead to complications including graft loss.

Patients undergo screening and diagnostic laboratory tests and imaging as necessary, specifically to exclude infection, malignancy, and chronic systemic disease. CT and MR angiography are used to study soft tissue, bony and vascular anatomy, to aid in producing 3D models,

---

Box 1
Care team

- Facial reconstruction and microsurgeons
- Physicians/Surgeons (transplant physicians, solid organ transplant surgeons, physical medicine and rehabilitation, oculoplastic surgeons, rhinologists, radiologist, infectious disease, dermatologist, pathologist, tissue typing, hematologist, immunologist, neurologist, among others).
- Speech therapist/pathologist
- Surgical technicians
- Administrators
- Ethicists
- Cadaver laboratory staff
- Illustrators
- Photographers
- Public relations personnel
- Visiting professors
- Biomedical engineers
- Organ Procurement Organization
- Physical and occupational therapist
- Regenerative medicine specialist
- Physician Assistants and Nurse Practitioners
- Transplant nurse coordinator
- Nurses
- Pharmacist
- Dentist
- Psychiatrist and addiction counselor
- Dietitian
- Social worker
- Anaplastologist

Box 2
Contraindications

Psychiatric
- Active psychiatric disorder
- Substance abuse

Psychosocial
- History of poor medical compliance
- Inadequate support system
- Pregnancy

Medical
- Blindness
- Hematologic/immunologic conditions: Hypercoagulable disorders, systemic lupus erythematosus, scleroderma
- Active or history of malignancy or high risk of cancer recurrence
- Active infectious disease (HIV, hepatitis)
- End-organ dysfunction

and to perform surgical planning. Electromyography (EMG) can be helpful in evaluating the function of facial muscles and nerves. After multidisciplinary discussion regarding the patient's eligibility, presurgical planning is performed, and the patient is placed on a waiting list. Candidates are reevaluated every few months to ensure updated medical history and screening. Donor criteria must consider sex, age, blood type and human leukocyte antigen (HLA) typing, panel reactive antibody testing, viral panels (eg, cytomegalovirus (CMV), Ebstein-Barr Virus (EBV), human immunodeficiency virus (HIV), hepatitis), body mass index, bony and soft tissue morphology, Fitzpatrick skin type matching,[18] and previous facial scars. For example, a suitable donor should have a similar Fitzpatrick skin type and depending on their age can be up to 20 years younger or 10 years older than the recipient.[19] When dealing with soft tissue size mismatch between the donor and recipient, our research on animal models demonstrated that fat transplanted responds to the surrounding microenvironment both macroscopically and microscopically, suggesting that transplantation of a face with an obesity mismatch would be acceptable.[20]

Immunologic Considerations

As with any allotransplantation, composite tissue allografts will be recognized as foreign by the recipient's immune system and will lead to immunologic rejection. The decision for facial transplantation over conventional reconstructive methods must be considered against the risks of lifelong immunosuppression, including shortened life expectancy due to complications of immunosuppression (such as increased risk of infectious complications, certain malignancies, and metabolic complications including posttransplant diabetes, renal failure, or even death).[21]

Preoperative Considerations

A transplant physician meets with the patient to discuss the immunosuppressive protocol and risks, monitoring, and potential complications. Conventional considerations in solid organ transplantation involve immunologic cross-reactivity and viral serology. In addition, face transplant candidates may be immunosensitized secondary to prior resuscitation with blood products or allogenic skin grafting.[22–24]

Immunosuppressive Regimen

Immunosuppressive therapy begins in the operating room (induction) and must continue (maintenance) lifelong with close monitoring. Induction is frequently achieved by lymphocyte-depleting agents such as antithymocyte globulin (ATG), which is a polyclonal antibody derived from rabbits directed against lymphocytes or monoclonal alemtuzumab that is directed against CD52 that is present on lymphocytes among other cells. A few transplants have been accomplished with a non–T-cell-depleting agent, basiliximab, that transiently blocks the interleukin-2 receptor α-chain (IL-2Rα, also known as CD25 antigen) on the surface of activated T-lymphocytes. Some cases have included the addition of anti-CD20 agent (Rituximab) aiming to specifically deplete B cells. These agents are combined with corticosteroids and followed by maintenance therapy that frequently consists of triple therapy comprising a calcineurin inhibitor (commonly tacrolimus - which prevents IL-2–dependent activation of lymphocytes), mycophenolate mofetil or mycophenolate sodium (antiproliferative agents), and varying doses of corticosteroids. In some cases, an mTOR inhibitor was substituted for the calcineurin inhibitor and in others, belatacept (a costimulation blocker) was used. Some centers have attempted experimental regimens to reduce the need for immunosuppression such as the use of unmodified donor bone marrow infusions, or mesenchymal stem cells.

Antimicrobial prophylaxis is frequently initiated at transplant and continues for varying durations; bacterial prophylaxis with trimethoprim-sulfamethoxazole for the prevention of Pneumocystis carinii and hardware infections, and viral prophylaxis with valganciclovir for the prevention of CMV are commonly used.[25] Antifungal prophylaxis is also frequently used. Side effects of immunosuppressives include steroid-induced diabetes mellitus, metabolic derangements (such as hyperglycemia and hyperlipidemia), hypertension, and renal toxicity.[26]

Rejection

Rejection, both acute and chronic, can result in transplant loss. Skin is considered the most antigenic of all the components of a composite allograft.[27] Almost all face transplant recipients reported in the literature have experienced an episode of acute rejection within a year postoperatively. Symptoms of acute rejection often manifest as cutaneous changes, such as erythema, edema, cutaneous rash, or mucosal lesions, and are graded using the Banff classification system, which is based on epithelial involvement and inflammatory cell infiltration.[28,29] Face transplant recipients should be closely monitored for signs of rejection, and treatment of rejection episodes must be initiated early (typically with pulse dose corticosteroids and adjustment of maintenance regimen). Steroid-resistant rejection requires the use of additional medications or plasmapheresis. In facial transplantation, there have been no reports of hyperacute rejection or graft-versus-host disease. Chronic rejection can be characterized by fibrotic changes, skin atrophy, dyschromias, telangiectasia, and skin sclerosis to full necrosis.[30] Classic perivascular graft rejection has been documented in cases of chronic rejection.[31] The cellular mechanisms underlying chronic rejection in facial transplantation are not fully understood, and may be T-cell mediated, B-cell mediated, or antibody mediated.[32,33] Furthermore, there is no consensus on managing these complications.

Sentinel flap

Sentinel flaps and routine skin and mucosal surveillance biopsies can also assist with clinical monitoring. The sentinel flap has the advantage of avoiding frequent serial biopsies to the facial allograft which can pose an esthetic concern.[34] In our case, a posterior tibial artery sentinel flap was used because of its reliable vascular pedicle, ease of harvest, and location away from the solid organ teams, thus enabling concurrent procurement. The flap was inset into the groin region for regular immune monitoring.

Salvage

Appropriate salvage options and backup plans are needed. The first facial retransplantation was performed by Lantieri and his team in France for a patient who underwent a face transplant in 2010 for neurofibromatosis. In 2016, the patient demonstrated signs of chronic rejection and complete graft excision was performed. A successful second transplantation was performed in 2018. In 2020, a second retransplantation was performed in Boston by Pomohac and his team. The patient received her first allotransplant in 2013 after burn injuries and demonstrated chronic rejection by 2019.[35]

Ethical Considerations

The foundational ethical principles of autonomy, beneficence, and nonmaleficence should be considered in every case. Unlike solid organ transplantation, facial transplantation is performed in patients with an otherwise normal life expectancy. Facial transplantation should only be considered in individuals who have suffered a loss of quality of life significant enough to accept the risks of lifelong immunosuppression and potential allograft rejection.[36] However, facial transplantation may help patients to regain their lost sense of identity, facilitate communication and social interactions

through facial expression, and enhance overall quality of life.[37–41]

Critics argue that self-identity may be altered in the setting of facial transplantation, including perceptions of identity to oneself and others, but loss of self-recognition is already likely present in many of these patients. Although full face transplants may look like donors in some features, variations in skeletal structure and soft tissue support in recipients assume a composite appearance distinct from donor or recipient. Nonetheless, in the United States, facial transplantation is approached as a separate donation decision from solid organ transplant because of the sensitivity of the procedure.[42,43] The transition to a new face is transformational and has been well-accepted. Most face transplants are performed as Institutional Review Board approved investigational clinical studies. Mayo Clinic performs VCA as an extension of clinical care with the program set up as a clinical program.

Informed consent must be considered, with particular populations being more vulnerable, such as patients with neurofibromatosis, blindness, and pediatrics.[44] Questions surrounding donor age and ethnicity mismatch and facial retransplantation have also been discussed.[45,46] Although face transplants have also been performed on patients with neurofibromatosis, concerns in these patients are the risk of transformation to neurofibrosarcoma once the immune system is compromised, and the risk of nerve involvement with tumor.[10,47] Early arguments questioned whether the benefits of a face transplant to a nonseeing individual would outweigh the risks of immunosuppression and extensive surgical reconstruction; however, facial transplantation has demonstrated increased interpersonal interaction and quality of life in this setting.[48–51] Facial transplantation in pediatric patients is also an ethical consideration, given that children do not have full autonomy to provide informed consent or the full capacity to perform a risk-benefit analysis of a life-long commitment to immunosuppression.[51] In a 2019 survey about opinions regarding facial transplantation, approximately 60% of polled ethicists agreed or strongly agreed that it could be permissible to perform a face transplant on a blind individual or child.[52]

Conventional reconstructive techniques are reviewed with the patient. For midfacial defects, this could include (1) staged nasal reconstruction with a free flap for inner nasal lining, cartilage grafts for structural support, and a forehead flap for outer nasal lining; (2) lip reconstruction with local flaps and a free functional gracilis flap; (3) oral restoration and staged dental rehabilitation which may include upper and lower jaw reconstruction with bone flaps, bony distraction, osseointegrated implants and prostheses. Complications associated with free tissue transfer are also reviewed, which may include wound healing complications, infection, hematoma, anesthetic complications, thrombosis, partial or total flap loss, among others.

Logistical Considerations

Optimizing workflow is critical for safe and efficient execution of these complex procedures. Collaboration with organ procurement organizations streamlines workflow processes for institutions to ensure team readiness. The team must be prepared to mobilize at any time. Simulations and cadaveric rehearsals allow the team to anticipate and to troubleshoot potential challenges, thereby refining workflows through repetition and outcomes assessments.

Conventional angiography and computerized tomographic angiography allow for visualization of vessel patency and flow dynamics in the head and neck, which is helpful for planning recipient dissection and graft procurement. 3D renderings provide information to assess both the donor and the recipient's skeletal anatomy.[53] 3D CT generated models and cutting guides, computer-aided design (CAD) and computer-aided manufacturing (CAM) and virtual surgical planning (VSP) can improve both planning and accuracy in craniofacial surgery and vascularized composite allotransplantation, and can increase efficiency and precision of donor and recipient osteotomies.[54–59]

In preparation for our first facial allotransplantation, we had simulation sessions with cadaveric dissections over 50 weekends. CTs of the donor and recipient were obtained, and cutting guides were created in collaboration with biomedical engineers from 3D Systems Inc. This technology allowed us to analyze cephalometric and occlusal relationships between donor and recipient craniomaxillofacial segments, and to analyze and refine outcomes for future cadaver sessions. Face transplant recipients often have challenging anatomy due to prior reconstructive attempts or complexities related to the initial defect. Utilization of VSP and 3D-printed positioning guides minimizes the impact of donor-recipient size mismatch and allows for precise inset and reconstruction with better facial esthetic and functional outcomes.[57–59] Intraoperative surgical navigation has also been proposed as an adjunct to improve accuracy of inset and fixation.

The current model involves 2 adjacent operating rooms, with teams working in parallel. In addition to the teams working on graft procurement and recipient preparation, a third team is performing procurement and transfer of the sentinel flap (free tissue transfer used to detect rejection episodes). The face transplant procurement is always done first before other solid organs are procured.[60] Forced breaks are instituted to keep members of the team functioning at the highest level and to help mitigate fatigue.

CASE

Facial transplantation integrates principles of plastic surgery, microsurgery, head and neck reconstruction, craniofacial surgery, orthognathics, facial esthetic surgery, and facial reanimation procedures.[61,62] For each recipient, the defect is carefully analyzed. When designing the facial allograft, functional and esthetic subunits are considered. The size and tissue components of the allograft are determined based on the soft tissue and bony defects.

At transplantation, our patient was a 31-year-old male with injury involving the face including the nose, zygomas, maxilla, and mandible, as well as facial soft tissue from the nasofrontal region to the neck. His history was significant for a self-inflicted gunshot wound to the face with multiple prior reconstructive procedures (Fig. 1).

Before facial transplantation, our patient had undergone vascularized free fibula for mandibular reconstruction and vascularized iliac for maxillary reconstruction and continued to have microstomia with difficulty eating, absence of the nose, and severe facial deformity. Even with these conventional reconstructive modalities, chewing would take him over 1 hour due to an absence of teeth. He was encumbered by breathing issues with his prosthetic nose, and desired to swim without aspirating. He also had to deal with the looks and comments of strangers, particularly children, when they saw his face. Considering further conventional facial reconstructive techniques which would involve multiple surgeries, a suboptimal outcome would be expected (Fig. 2). In phase 1, a nasal reconstruction with radial forearm flap, rib cartilage graft, and forehead flap would be performed. In phase 2, oral sphincter reconstruction and reanimation would involve multiple procedures, including a free gracilis and skin graft. In phase 3, midface retrusion would require horizontal distraction of the neomaxilla and placement of osseointegrated implants. The option of a face transplant would permit transfer of the structures below the eyelids, including the nose, maxilla, mandible, teeth, muscles of the face and skin, nerves, and blood vessels. VSP and 3D-printed cutting guides (Figs. 3 and 4) minimize the impact

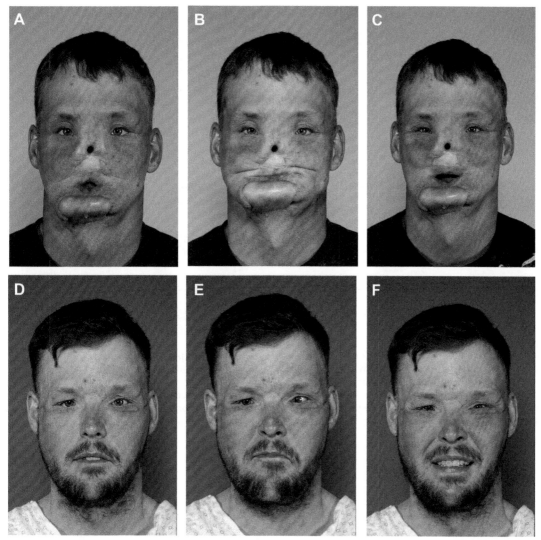

Fig. 1. Preoperative views (*A*) anterior in repose; (*B*) mouth closure; (*C*) smile Postoperative views (*D*) anterior in repose; (*E*) mouth closure; (*F*) smile. (Used with permission of Mayo Foundation for Medical Education and Research, all rights reserved.)

of donor-recipient size mismatches and allow for precise reconstruction with improved facial esthetic and functional outcomes.

Donor Procurement

Our preference is to use total intravenous anesthesia rather than inhalational anesthesia until all nerve branches have been identified and stimulated. Incisions should be planned to provide the most inconspicuous scarring. Individualized planning is crucial and esthetic subunits should be respected. Skin incisions are designed in the donor corresponding to the defect created in the recipient's face during preparation for transplant. Skin flaps are elevated from lateral to medial

beyond the parotid gland. A high superficial musculoaponeurotic system (SMAS) flap is elevated, and dissection continues anterior to where the nerve branches exit the parotid gland. The proximal facial nerve is then identified by dissecting down to the tragal pointer and locating the main trunk of the facial nerve posterior and inferior. The facial nerve is dissected from proximal to distal through the parotid gland and a superficial parotedectomy is performed. A photograph of the nerves is taken, stimulation of the nerves is performed and video recorded, and the functions of each branch is written on the printed photograph for later identification including smile, snarl, lower lip depression, and identification of the orbicularis oculi and oris muscles (**Fig. 5**). The

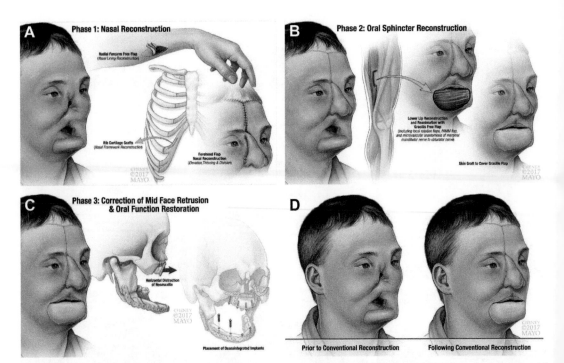

Fig. 2. Illustration depicting conventional facial reconstructive techniques. (*A*) Phase 1: Nasal reconstruction with radial forearm flap, rib cartilage graft, and forehead flap. (*B*) Phase 2: Oral sphincter reconstruction and reanimation with free gracilis and skin graft. (*C*) Phase 3: Correction of midface retrusion and oral function restoration with horizontal distraction of neomaxilla and placement of osseointegrated implants. (*D*) Before and following conventional reconstruction. (Used with permission of Mayo Foundation for Medical Education and Research, all rights reserved.)

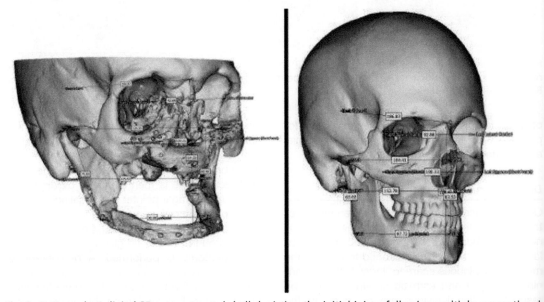

Fig. 3. Pretransplant digital 3D- reconstructed skull depicting the initial injury following multiple conventional reconstructive procedures, before transplant (left) and depicting the virtual surgical plan for the normative skull to be achieved during a transplant(right). (Used with permission of Mayo Foundation for Medical Education and Research, all rights reserved.)

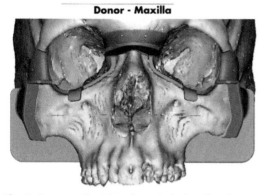
Donor - Maxilla

Fig. 4. Preoperative virtual surgical planning demonstrating donor cutting guides. (Used with permission of Mayo Foundation for Medical Education and Research, all rights reserved.)

proximal facial nerve is then dissected toward the stylomastoid foramen and cut.

The facial transplant is supplied by the facial artery and drained by the common facial vein on each side. The amount of tissue that is procured from the donor depends on the defect to be reconstructed in the recipient. In order to achieve optimal outcomes and produce inconspicuous scars, major units in the face need to be preserved. For example, when reconstructing complex midface defects, the scars are placed in the lower eyelids, across the radix, in the preauricular area, and across the neck. Neck dissection involves elevation of a subplatysmal flap and circumferential exposure of neurovascular structures such as the common, external, and internal carotid arteries; internal jugular vein; facial artery and vein; superficial temporal, internal maxillary, occipital, and lingual vessels; and hypoglossal nerve. The posterior belly of the digastric and hypoglossal nerve are cut. The common facial vein is then identified and dissected proximally and included along with a segment of the internal jugular vein. The facial vessels supply the entire flap. Timing of transection of the vessels is coordinated closely with the recipient defect preparation to minimize ischemia time. The same procedure is performed on the contralateral side. **Fig. 5**. Sensory nerves depending on the anatomic structures transferred (eg, infraorbital, supraorbital, supratrochlear, and inferior alveolar) are identified and transected proximally to provide length for coaptation to the recipient sensory nerves following bony inset (**Fig. 1**). The masseter is then removed from the lateral aspect of the mandible.

Then, cutting guides are placed onto the mandible, marking the area where we would resect the condyle and coronoid to provide

exposure to the pterygomaxillary junction and inferior alveolar nerve, lingual nerve, and sensory nerve to the buccal mucosa, cutting these proximally and tagging for later identification. Then, the zygoma, lateral orbital rim, and zygomatic arch osteotomy sites are exposed. The attachment of the facial muscles to the zygoma body are maintained and all tissue lateral and superior to the areas of osteotomies are dissected off the bone. Soft tissues attachments to the ramus and body of the mandible are separated from the bone and cutting guides are placed. The same is performed on the contralateral side and the soft tissues overlying the nasofrontal region are elevated off of the bone. The infraorbital rim, orbital floor, and infraorbital nerve are also identified. Osteotomy guides are placed on the nasofrontal region, zygomas bilaterally, and mandibles bilaterally and secured in place. Then, a sagittal bone saw or PiezoElectric saw (DePuy Synthes, Raynham, MA) is used to perform a LeFort III osteotomy and disimpaction as well as a sagittal split osteotomy. When upper and lower jaws are included in the transplant, oral mucosa, inner cheek mucosa, hard palate, and some soft palate are included in the donor procurement. The muscle attachment from the neck to the mandible are elevated off the bone except for a small area anteriorly where the tendineos portion is kept attached to the bone so that the recipient's anterior neck muscles are reattached to the transplanted mandible. Disimpaction of the LeFort III segment is performed. The neck vessels are clamped and the vessels are cut at the external carotid and internal jugular levels bilaterally and flushed with heparinized saline. The transplant is taken to the recipient room for organ donation. In collaboration with anaplastologists, silicone or resin masks can be handcrafted or 3D printed to restore the congruency of the donor site and allow for an "open casket" burial.[63]

Recipient Preparation

Open tracheostomy and percutaneous endoscopic gastrostomy tube placement are performed. For midfacial reconstructions including the upper and lower jaw and soft tissues, the incisions are marked at the nasofrontal junction,eyelid-cheek junction, and then crossing over to the preauricular, and submandibularregions bilaterally. An incision is made in the nasolabial crease bilaterally. Skin flaps are dissected from medial to lateral in the subcutaneous plane to allow for exposure and dissection of the facial nerve branches distal to the parotid gland, and identification of the function of each branch

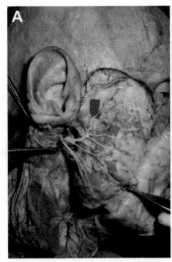
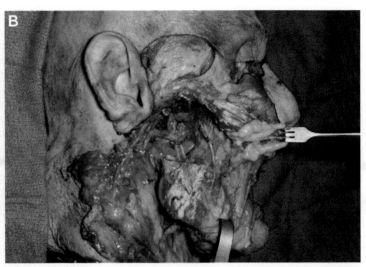

Fig. 5. Cadaveric dissections of facial nerves (*A*) and proximal segment of mandible removed allowing for visualization of the inferior alveolar, lingual, and sensory branch supplying the buccal mucosa (*B*). (Used with permission of Mayo Foundation for Medical Education and Research, all rights reserved.)

through nerve stimulation. Furthermore, this allows for preservation of perforators to the skin in the preauricular region in the event that procurement is aborted because of donor instability, so in that case the skin flaps can be repositioned and closed. Facial nerve branches are all identified and marked for their function with different sutures. Recipient vessels including external carotid and facial vessels are identified in the neck.

The recipient facial nerves are transected distal to the parotid gland and dissected from medial to lateral to allow for exposure of the underlying skeleton. The zygoma, lateral orbital rim, mandible and pterygomaxillary junction are exposed. The mandible is dissected free from the surrounding soft tissues and the proximal segment of the mandible is fixated in position to the zygomatic arches with guides to allow for the proximal segment to be in the proper position when insetting the donor face.

Once it is deemed that the donor is stable and solid organ teams can wait to procure organs, custom-tailored virtually designed 3D-printed surgical guides are then affixed at the planned LeFort III bony osteotomies including the zygomas, lateral orbital rims, nasofrontal region, junction of the pterygoid with the prior iliac bone, and sagittal splits of the mandible bilaterally.

The LeFort III segment is disimpacted then areas of bony prominence on the recipient defect are then assessed and rongeured to correct the contour needed to best fit the donor graft. 3D-printed "fit guides" aid in determining whether there are bony prominences in the recipient defect. The donor graft is then brought into the

field, and bony fixation is performed. In our case, we secured the zygoma of the donor to the zygomatic arches of the recipient bilaterally and the lateral orbital rim as well as the nasofrontal region and secured the mandible with screws. Microvascular anatomosis of the recipient arteries and veins of the donor and recipient are performed.

Neurorrhaphies of the facial nerve branches are performed. The SMAS is then positioned at appropriate tension and sutured in place. The lacrimal sacs are sutured and pigtail stents are placed to assure patency of the canaliculi during healing in collaboration with oculoplastics team (**Fig. 6**). On both sides, the patient's telecanthus is repaired by suturing his native medial canthal tendon and medial orbital tissue to the firmly adherent tissue of the donor medial orbital wall.

The parotid ducts are stented using lacrimal probes, and a silastic tubing is used to intubate the proximal and distal ends of the parotid ducts, which are repaired over the stents using interrupted nylon sutures. The silastic stents are secured to the buccal mucosa and removed 2 weeks post operatively.

Considerations

Vasculature
Facial transplantation involves *en bloc* replacement of tissues, and requires careful consideration of blood supply. Vessel selection is dependent upon the tissues transplanted and the defect to be reconstructed.[64,65] Angiography and clinical experience demonstrate that the facial artery is sufficient to supply a full face transplant including

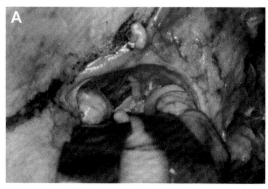 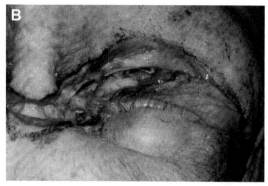

Fig. 6. Proximal dissection of orbital floor and infraorbital nerves (*A*) and lacrimal system (*B*). (Used with permission of Mayo Foundation for Medical Education and Research, all rights reserved.)

the upper and lower eyelids, maxilla anterior to the pterygoids, anterior portion of the mandible, nose, and lips. The palate, while primarily supplied by the palatine vessels from the internal maxillary system, can be perfused by the oral mucosal vasculature from the facial artery. In our anatomic dissections, we found it feasible to dissect the internal maxillary artery to the point where it supplies the maxilla, however, osteotomies often preclude inclusion of the vessel branches. While the scalp and lateral face are supplied by the superficial temporal artery, the facial artery can supply the entire facial allograft. To include the entire scalp, the posterior occipital should be included. In a few described cases, the external carotid has been used. The external carotid can be used for the donor tissue if the internal maxillary vessels, superficial temporal or posterior occipital vessels are needed to supply a larger portion of the facial soft tissue or bony skeleton. The venous outflow is often based on the common facial veins. Allograft perfusion and viability after vascular anastomoses can be verified using indocyanine green fluorescence angiography if needed.

Nerves
Face transplant success is highly dependent on regeneration of the facial nerve, leading to restoration of facial movement and function.[66] Goals include restoration of spontaneous and symmetric facial movement, smile, and emotional expression. A "mask-like" appearance is expected for several months until facial nerve regeneration occurs, which is estimated at a rate of 1 mm of nerve regeneration to the distal target daily. Nerve coaptation follows bony fixation and allograft revascularization. Motor function is restored by performing neurorrhaphy between the donor and recipient's facial nerve, either distally at the level of the facial nerve branches or proximally at the

level of the facial nerve trunk. To achieve the best functional outcomes, coaptation of motor nerves to the eyelids, upper lip, commissure, and lower lip are performed to achieve blink, speech, and swallowing. A superficial parotidectomy on the donor allows identification of the facial nerve branches within the parotid gland and minimizes bulk of the cheeks. Tension-free neurorrhaphies of donor and recipient branches with identical function are performed using the prior functional assessment of each branch motor function.[67,68]

Coaptation location of the donor and recipient facial nerves is a subject of controversy. Proximal coaptation of the facial trunk simplifies neurorrhaphy technique and decreases operative time. Dividing the facial nerve distally can result in creation of unexpected gaps when nerve coaptation is performed between the recipient's and donor's facial nerves. Our group prefers distal facial nerve coaptation to minimize aberrant reinnervation and synkinesis, and to facilitate functional recovery given the short distance the nerve fibers need to regenerate to reach target muscles. This requires facial nerve mapping of individual nerve branches using an intraoperative nerve stimulator, which we suggest performing while the face is video recorded so that muscle movement can be carefully assessed and the ideal nerve branches in donor and recipient can be matched (see **Fig. 3**). Coaptation of sensory nerves leads to more predictable reinnervation and protection of donor tissue and thus should be performed whenever possible. Depending on the type of face transplant, coaptation of the supraorbital, infraorbital, inferior alveolar, and mental nerves are performed to aid in sensory restoration. Proximal dissection of the donor nerve and distal dissection of the recipient nerve allow for sensory nerve coaptation to be performed following bony fixation at the level of the orbital rim for the infraorbital nerve and below the mandible border for the inferior alveolar nerve. Sensory recovery has been reported in patients for whom sensory nerve coaptation was not performed, likely from regeneration of surrounding nerve fibers.[69]

Postoperatively, it is also important to initiate biofeedback-driven facial reanimation therapy and neuromuscular rehabilitation early, and to address synkinesis through mirror feedback and retraining therapy.

Soft tissue

Finally, all soft tissue is approximated and closed. The intraoral soft tissue is approximated including the oral floor, soft palate and posterior cheek. Salivary gland management has been debated.[70] Some allotransplants include both superficial and deep parotid lobes, some only the superficial lobe, and some exclude the entire gland. Transplanting the entire parotid gland has the benefit of reducing operative time and minimizing the possibility of damage to the facial nerve, but fistula, sialocele, bulky appearance, and wound healing complications may ensue. The recipient is then placed in mandibulomaxillary fixation with rubber bands.

Outcomes

Outcomes in facial transplantation are not standardized because of the limited number of procedures performed globally. It is difficult to accurately estimate complication rates because of the unique characteristics of each patient's injuries including preoperative functional status, varied allograft flap design and technical aspects, individualized immunosuppressive regimens and graft surveillance protocols, and the lack of standardized or validated reporting measures.[71] Systematic reviews have demonstrated that facial transplantation leads to an improved quality of life and functional outcomes.[72] Reported outcomes are often divided into functional (breathing, eating, speaking), aesthetic, immunologic, and psychosocial. Development and sharing of validated protocols is essential to improve patient outcomes and to maximize the results of this procedure.[73]

Facial tracking technologies and video analysis have been used to track recovery of facial expression and speech. Motor recovery occurred for most patients between 6 and 18 months, including improvement in breathing, speaking, and facial movement, and removal of feeding tubes and decannulation when initially present. Return of facial motor function following proximal facial nerve repair revealed higher rates of synkinesis, and resulted in repair of facial nerve branches distally to reduce the distance to target muscles.[69,74–77] Previously published outcomes data assess the

level of facial nerve coaptation, time to return of facial motor function, EMG studies, and development of synkinesis. Thermal and pressure sensation have been reported at 2 weeks and 6 months after transplantation, respectively. Thus far, 7 face transplant recipients have died; causes of death include medication noncompliance, infection, malignancy, and suicide.

Dental, Speech, and Swallowing Outcomes

Dental restoration and rehabilitation in face transplant recipients is important to optimization of occlusion and overall health. Postoperative occlusion correction can include orthodontics, dental prosthetics, and orthognathic surgery. A speech and language pathologist is part of the face transplant team and helps guide speech therapy following transplant. Reported outcomes should include word production, intelligibility, voice, resonance, speech acceptability, and articulation.

Revisions

Revision surgeries are often necessary following facial transplantation to achieve optimal functional and esthetic outcomes. Intraoperative and immediate postoperative assessments are often difficult to perform due to edema. Malocclusion may be present because of allograft discrepancies or unstable skeletal movement and may require surgical or nonsurgical correction. Scar revision, soft tissue or ligamentous resuspension, and/or debulking may need to be performed. Data on posttransplant revisions is lacking, but it is important to discuss that these procedures may be performed to improve functional and aesthetic outcomes and to address postoperative complications such as enophthalmos, ptosis, ectropion, malocclusion, palatal fistulae, and contour abnormalities.[78,79]

SUMMARY

The midface is the foundation for human social, communicative, and emotional function, and is essential to facial identity that is consequently the basis of human relationships. Facial transplantation is a vascularized composite allotransplantation which may be considered in patients with extensive and challenging facial defects for which conventional reconstructive approaches fail to provide satisfactory functional and esthetic outcomes. Facial VCA can be considered as the highest rung on the reconstructive ladder and provides an option to restore the face in appearance and function in a single surgery. Success is reliant on patient understanding, motivation, consent, compliance, and a multidisciplinary approach with careful team planning and organization. At our institution, each step of the procedure was performed and refined over a series of cadaver dissections. Preparation was further optimized with the use of VSP and cutting guides. Specific attention must be provided to skeletal positioning, dental occlusion, and nerve coaptation. The decision for facial transplantation over conventional reconstructive methods must be considered against the risks of lifelong immunosuppression. Facial transplantation will constantly evolve because of a combination of multidisciplinary advances. Future goals in VCA should include research in tolerance induction and reducing adverse effects associated with immunosuppression. It is difficult to accurately estimate complication rates and compare outcomes due to the small number of cases, unique characteristics of each patient's injuries, and varied regimens employed. Sharing experiences and outcomes data is essential to further improve results.

DISCLOSURE

The authors have nothing to disclose.

REFERENCES

1. Rifkin WJ, David JA, Plana NM, et al. Achievements and challenges in facial transplantation. Ann Surg 2018;268(2):260–70.
2. Coffman KL, Gordon C, Siemionow M. Psychological outcomes with face transplantation: overview and case report. Curr Opin Organ Transplant 2010; 15(2):236–40.
3. Devauchelle B, Badet L, Lengelé B, et al. First human face allograft: early report. Lancet 2006; 368(9531):203–9.
4. Meningaud JP, Hivelin M, Benjoar MD, et al. The procurement of allotransplants for ballistic trauma: a preclinical study and a report of two clinical cases. Plast Reconstr Surg 2011;127(5):1892–900.
5. Pomahac B, Pribaz J, Eriksson E, et al. Restoration of facial form and function after severe disfigurement from burn injury by a composite facial allograft. Am J Transplant 2011;11(2):386–93.
6. Pomahac B, Pribaz J, Eriksson E, et al. Three patients with full facial transplantation. N Engl J Med 2012;366(8):715–22.
7. Roche NA, Vermeersch HF, Stillaert FB, et al. Complex facial reconstruction by vascularized composite allotransplantation: the first Belgian case. J Plast Reconstr Aesthet Surg 2015;68(3): 362–71.
8. Siemionow MZ, Papay F, Djohan R, et al. First U.S. near-total human face transplantation: a paradigm shift for massive complex injuries. Plast Reconstr Surg 2010;125(1):111–22.
9. Siemionow M. The decade of face transplant outcomes. J Mater Sci Mater Med 2017;28(5):64.
10. Krakowczyk L, Maciejewski A, Szymczyk C, et al. Face transplant in an advanced neurofibromatosis type 1 patient. Ann Transplant 2017;22:53–7.
11. Gomez-Cia T, Sicilia-Castro D, Infante-Cossio P, et al. Second human facial allotransplantation to restore a severe defect following radical resection of bilateral massive plexiform neurofibromas. Plast Reconstr Surg 2011;127(2):995–6.
12. Lantieri L, Meningaud JP, Grimbert P, et al. Repair of the lower and middle parts of the face by composite tissue allotransplantation in a patient with massive plexiform neurofibroma: a 1-year follow-up study. Lancet 2008;372(9639):639–45.
13. Sosin M, Rodriguez ED. The face transplantation update: 2016. Plast Reconstr Surg 2016;137(6): 1841–50.
14. Losee JE, Fletcher DR, Gorantla VS. Human facial allotransplantation: patient selection and pertinent considerations. J Craniofac Surg 2012;23(1): 260–4.
15. Pomahac B, Diaz-Siso JR, Bueno EM. Evolution of indications for facial transplantation. J Plast Reconstr Aesthet Surg 2011;64(11):1410–6.
16. Dahlborg EJ, Diaz-Siso JR, Bueno EM, et al. The value of innovation: face and hand transplantation programs at Brigham and Women's Hospital. Plast Reconstr Surg 2014;134(1):178e–9e.
17. Soni CV, Barker JH, Pushpakumar SB, et al. Psychosocial considerations in facial transplantation. Burns 2010;36:959–64.
18. Bueno E, Diaz-Siso J, Pomahac B. A multidisciplinary protocol for face transplantation at Brigham and Women's Hospital. J Plast Reconstr Aesthet Surg 2011;64(12):1572–9.
19. Aflaki P, Nelson C, Balas B, et al. Simulated central face transplantation: age consideration in matching donors and recipients. J Plast Reconstr Aesthet Surg 2010;63(3):e283–5.
20. Suchyta M, Gibreel W, Bakri K, et al. Transplanted fat adapts to the environment of the recipient: an animal study using a murine model to investigate the suitability of recipient obesity mismatch in face transplantation. J Plast Reconstr Aesthet Surg 2020;73(1):176–83.
21. Chim H, Amer H, Mardini S, et al. Vascularized composite allotransplant in the realm of regenerative plastic surgery [published correction appears in Mayo Clin Proc. 2014 Aug;89(8):1169]. Mayo Clin Proc 2014;89(7):1009–20.
22. Ng ZY, Lellouch AG, Drijkoningen T, et al. Vascularized composite allotransplantation-an emerging

concept for burn reconstruction. J Burn Care Res 2017;38:371–8.

23. Brandacher G. Composite tissue transplantation. Methods Mol Biol 2013;1034:103–15.

24. Kueckelhaus M, Fischer S, Seyda M, et al. Vascularized composite allotransplantation: current standards and novel approaches to prevent acute rejection and chronic allograft deterioration. Transpl Int 2016;29(06):655–62.

25. Razonable RR, Amer H, Mardini S. Application of a New Paradigm for Cytomegalovirus Disease Prevention in Mayo Clinic's First Face Transplant. Mayo Clin Proc 2019;94(1):166–70.

26. Lantieri L, Grimbert P, Ortonne N, et al. Face transplant: long-term follow-up and results of a prospective open study. Lancet 2016;388(10052):1398–407.

27. Lee WP, Yaremchuk MJ, Pan YC, et al. Relative antigenicity of components of a vascularized limb allograft. Plast Reconstr Surg 1991;87(03):401–11.

28. Cendales L, Kanitakis J, Schneeberger S, et al. The Banff 2007 working classification of skin containing composite tissue allograft pathology. Am J Transplant 2008;8(7):1396–400.

29. Sis B, Mengel M, Haas M, et al. Banff'09 meeting report: antibody mediated graft deterioration and implementation of Banff working groups. Am J Transplant 2010;10(3):464–71.

30. Morelon E, Petruzzo P, Kanitakis J, et al. Face transplantation: Partial graft loss of the first case 10 years later. Am J Transplant 2017;17:1935–40.

31. Petruzzo P, Kanitakis J, Testelin S, et al. Clinicopathological findings of chronic rejection in a face grafted patient. Transplantation 2015;99(12):2644–50.

32. Kaufman CL, Cascalho M, Ozyurekoglu T, et al. The role of B cell immunity in VCA graft rejection and acceptance. Hum Immunol 2019;80(06):385–92.

33. Lee ZH, Lopez CD, Plana NM, et al. Are we prepared for the inevitable? A survey on defining and managing failure in face transplantation. Plast Reconstr Surg Glob Open 2019;7(05):e2055.

34. Kueckelhaus M, Fischer S, Lian CG, et al. Utility of sentinel flaps in assessing facial allograft rejection. Plast Reconstr Surg 2015;135(1):250–8.

35. Kauke M, Panayi AC, Safi AF, et al. Full facial re-transplantation in a female patient-Technical, immunologic, and clinical considerations. Am J Transplant 2021;21(10):3472–80.

36. Barker JH, Brown CS, Cunningham M, et al. Ethical considerations in human facial tissue allotransplantation. Ann Plast Surg 2008;60(1):103–9.

37. Alam D, Papay F, Djohan R. Technical and anatomical aspects of the world's first near total face and maxilla transplant. Arch Facial Plast Surg 2009; 11(6):369–77.

38. Kiwanuka H, Bueno EM, Diaz-Siso JR, et al. Evolution of ethical debate on face transplantation. Plast Reconstr Surg 2013;132(6):1558–68.

39. Rifkin WJ, Kantar RS, Ali-Khan S, et al. Facial disfigurement and identity: a review of the literature and implications for facial transplantation. AMA J Ethics 2018;20(4):309–23.

40. Aycart MA, Kiwanuka H, Krezdorn N, et al. Quality of life after face transplantation: outcomes, assessment tools, and future directions. Plast Reconstr Surg 2017;139(1):194–203.

41. Taylor-Alexander S. Unmaking responsibility: patient death and face transplantation. Curr Anthropol 2016;57(4):511–6.

42. Coffman KL, Siemionow MZ. Ethics of facial transplantation revisited. Curr Opin Organ Transplant 2014;19(2):181–7.

43. Butler PE, Hettiaratchy S, Clarke A. Managing the risks of facial transplantation. Lancet 2006;368: 561–3.

44. Devauchelle BL, Testelin SR, Davrou J, et al. Face graft? Extrapolation of facial allotransplantation to children. J Craniomaxillofac Surg 2016;44(8): 925–33.

45. Theodorakopoulou E, Meghji S, Pafitanis G, et al. A review of the world's published face transplant cases: ethical perspectives. Scars Burn Heal 2017; 3. 2059513117694402.

46. Siemionow M, Ozturk C. Face transplantation: outcomes, concerns, controversies, and future directions. J Craniofac Surg 2012;23(1):254–9.

47. Sicilia-Castro D, Gomez-Cia T, Infante-Cossio P, et al. Reconstruction of a severe facial defect by allotransplantation in neurofibromatosis type 1: a case report. Transplant Proc 2011;43(7):2831–7.

48. Bramstedt KA, Plock JA. Looking the world in the face: the benefits and challenges of facial transplantation for blind patients. Prog Transplant 2017;27(1): 79–83.

49. Carty MJ, Bueno EM, Lehmann LS, et al. A position paper in support of face transplantation in the blind. Plast Reconstr Surg 2012;130(2):319–24.

50. Hendrickx H, Blondeel PN, Van Parys H, et al. Facing a new face: an interpretative phenomenological analysis of the experiences of a blind face transplant patient and his partner. J Craniofac Surg 2018;29(4): 826–31.

51. Marchac A, Kuschner T, Paris J, et al. Ethical issues in pediatric face transplantation: should we perform face transplantation in children? Plast Reconstr Surg 2016;138(2):449–54.

52. Suchyta MA, Sharp R, Amer H, et al. Ethicists' opinions regarding the permissibility of face transplant. Plast Reconstr Surg 2019;144(1):212–24.

53. Suchyta M, Mardini S. Innovations and future directions in head and neck microsurgical reconstruction. Clin Plast Surg 2017;44(2):325–44.

54. Chim H, Wetjen N, Mardini S. Virtual surgical planning in craniofacial surgery. Semin Plast Surg 2014;28(3):150–8.

55. Zhao L, Patel PK, Cohen M. Application of virtual surgical planning with computer assisted design and manufacturing technology to cranio-maxillofacial surgery. Arch Plast Surg 2012;39(4):309–16.

56. Rodby KA, Turin S, Jacobs RJ, et al. Advances in oncologic head and neck reconstruction: systematic review and future considerations of virtual surgical planning and computer aided design/computer aided modeling. J Plast Reconstr Aesthet Surg 2014;67(9):1171–85.

57. Dorafshar AH, Brazio PS, Mundinger GS, et al. Found in space: computer-assisted orthognathic alignment of a total face allograft in six degrees of freedom. J Oral Maxillofac Surg 2014;72(09):1788–800.

58. Brown EN, Dorafshar AH, Bojovic B, et al. Total face, double jaw, and tongue transplant simulation: a cadaveric study using computer-assisted techniques. Plast Reconstr Surg 2012;130(4):815–23.

59. Hashemi S, Armand M, Gordon CR. Development and refinement of computer-assisted planning and execution system for use in face-jaw-teeth transplantation to improve skeletal and dento-occlusal outcomes. Curr Opin Organ Transplant 2016;21(5):523–9.

60. Petruzzo P, Testelin S, Kanitakis J, et al. First human face transplantation: 5 years outcomes. Transplantation 2012;93:236–40.

61. Pomahac B, Bueno EM, Sisk GC, et al. Current principles of facial allotransplantation: the Brigham and Women's Hospital Experience. Plast Reconstr Surg 2013;131(5):1069–76.

62. Sosin M, Ceradini DJ, Hazen A, et al. Total face, eyelids, ears, scalp, and skeletal subunit transplant cadaver simulation: the culmination of aesthetic, craniofacial, and microsurgery principles. Plast Reconstr Surg 2016;137(5):1569–81.

63. Grant GT, Liacouras P, Santiago GF, et al. Restoration of the donor face after facial allotransplantation: digital manufacturing techniques. Ann Plast Surg 2014;72(6):720–4.

64. Pomahac B, Lengele B, Ridgway EB, et al. Vascular considerations in composite midfacial allotransplantation. Plast Reconstr Surg 2010;125:517–22.

65. Pomahac B, Gobble RM, Schneeberger S. Facial and hand allotransplantation. Cold Spring Harbor Perspect Med 2014;4(3):a015651.

66. Arun A, Abt NB, Tuffaha S, et al. Nerve regeneration in vascularized composite allotransplantation: current strategies and future directions. Plast Aesthet Res 2015;2:226–35.

67. Ray WZ, Mackinnon SE. Management of nerve gaps: autografts, allografts, nerve transfers, and end-to-side neurorrhaphy. Exp Neurol 2010;223(1):77–85.

68. Bassilios Habre S, Bond G, Jing XL, et al. The surgical management of nerve gaps: present and future. Ann Plast Surg 2018;80(3):252–61.

69. Siemionow M, Gharb BB, Rampazzo A. Pathways of sensory recovery after face transplantation. Plast Reconstr Surg 2011;127(5):1875–89.

70. Frautschi R, Rampazzo A, Bernard S, et al. Management of the salivary glands and facial nerve in face transplantation. Plast Reconstr Surg 2016;137(06):1887–97.

71. Aycart MA, Kiwanuka H, Krezdorn N, et al. Quality of life after face transplantation: Outcomes, assessment tools, and future directions. Plast Reconstr Surg 2017;139:194–203.

72. Fischer S, Kueckelhaus M, Pauzenberger R, et al. Functional outcomes of face transplantation. Am J Transplant 2015;15(1):220–33.

73. Daneshgaran G, Stern CS, Garfein ES. Reporting practices on immunosuppression and rejection management in face transplantation: A systematic review. J Reconstr Microsurg 2019;35(9):652–61.

74. Pomahac B, Pribaz JJ, Bueno EM, et al. Novel surgical technique for full face transplantation. Plast Reconstr Surg 2012;130(3):549–55.

75. Aycart MA, Perry B, Alhefzi M, et al. Surgical optimization of motor recovery in face transplantation. J Craniofac Surg 2016;27(2):286–92.

76. Khalifian S, Brazio PS, Mohan R, et al. Facial transplantation: the first 9 years. Lancet 2014;384(9960):2153–63.

77. Lantieri L, Hivelin M, Audard V, et al. Feasibility, reproducibility, risks and benefits of face transplantation: a prospective study of outcomes. Am J Transplant 2011;11(2):367–78.

78. Mohan R, Fisher M, Dorafshar A, et al. Principles of face transplant revision: beyond primary repair. Plast Reconstr Surg 2014;134(6):1295–304.

79. Aycart MA, Alhefzi M, Kueckelhaus M, et al. A retrospective analysis of secondary revisions after face transplantation: assessment of outcomes, safety, and feasibility. Plast Reconstr Surg 2016;138(4):690e–701e.

Facial Recognition Pattern before and after Lower Eyelid Blepharoplasty
An Eye Tracking Analysis

Francesco Bernardini, MD[a,1], Tim Staiger[b,1], Nicholas Moellhoff, MD[b],
Riccardo E. Giunta, MD[b], David Braig, MD, PhD[b], Denis Ehrl, MD, PhD[b],
Julie Woodward, MD[c], Sebastian Cotofana, MD, PhD[d], Lukas H. Kohler, MD[b],
Konstantin Frank, MD[b,*]

KEYWORDS

• Facial recognition • Periorbital anatomy • Blepharoplasty • Eye tracking analyses • Facial anatomy

INTRODUCTION

According to the International Society of Aesthetic Plastic Surgeons a total of 1.3 million eyelid surgery procedures were performed in 2019, indicating an increase of 14.5% compared with 2018.[1] Although injections of soft tissue fillers in the lower orbital region have gained popularity, periorbital surgery is required in many instances to provide a sufficient and successful long-term result. With increasing age, the bony orbit, the ligaments, the subcutaneous fat, the muscle, and the skin undergo significant changes that cause an accentuation of the tear trough, infraorbital hollowing, herniation of the intraorbital fat pads, excess upper and lower lid skin, festoons, and eyelid hooding.[2–8] Age-related changes and the resulting clinical manifestations in the periorbital region often lead to a tired and unhappy facial expression. Because the eyes are considered as the center of attention and are often looked on first when observing a face, age-related changes in this area might be more visible and apparent than other characteristics of an aged face. Aesthetic periocular surgery aims to ameliorate or even mask these signs of aging, thereby creating a younger, fresher, and more harmonious look.[9] Although patient-reported and physician-reported outcome are valuable when it comes to assessing the success of aesthetic facial surgery, eye tracking technology has emerged as a novel technique and method to assess the gaze of participants when looking at bodies. Recent investigations have shown that people tend to look faster and longer at facial characteristics that seem unharmonious and disproportionate[10,11] Altering the periorbital appearance of a patient might thus consecutively change the facial feature sequence of observers. Signs of aging, which might capture the gaze and look of a viewer before periorbital surgery, might be looked at longer and quicker because they might be perceived as unharmonious, whereas the face and especially the periorbital region of patients that underwent periorbital cosmetic surgery might be viewed differently after amelioration or masking of aforementioned signs

Author disclosure: The authors declared no potential conflicts of interest with respect to the research, authorship, and publication of this article.
Funding: The authors received no financial support for the research, authorship, and publication of this article.
[a] Oculoplastica Bernardini, Genova, Italy; [b] Department for Hand, Plastic and Aesthetic Surgery, Ludwig – Maximilian University Munich, Munich, Germany; [c] Duke University Medical Center, Durham, NC, USA; [d] Department of Clinical Anatomy, Mayo Clinic College of Medicine and Science, Rochester, MN, USA
[1] Both authors contributed equally.
* Corresponding author: Department for Hand, Plastic and Aesthetic Surgery Ludwig – Maximilian University Munich, Pettenkoferstraße 8A, Munich 80336, Germany.
E-mail address: konstantinfrank@me.com

of aging. Thus, the aim of this study was to investigate eye movement patterns using eye tracking technology when looking at preoperative and postoperative images of patients that underwent bilateral periorbital cosmetic surgery.

MATERIAL AND METHODS
Study Sample

This study investigated the eye movement pattern of 58 volunteers with a mean age of 37.0 ± 15.8 years, of which 21 were males (36.2%) and 37 females (63.8%). Volunteers were recruited, of which 12 (20.7%) were plastic surgeons and 46 (79.3%) were without medical background.

Before enrollment, volunteers consented for the use of their demographic and result-related data for the purposes of this study. The investigation was institutional review board approved (protocol number: 20–1018). This study was conducted in accordance with regional laws and good clinical practice, and in accordance with the Declaration of Helsinki.[12] Patients gave their informed consent for their images to be published.

Eye Movement Analyses

The investigations of eye movements were conducted with eye tracking technology and as described previously.[13] In brief, the gaze pattern of the included volunteers was investigated using a Tobii Pro Nano eye tracker (Tobii Pro AB, Stockholm, Sweden) with a frequency of 60 Hz. The eye-tracker bar was fixed to a 15-inch screen (339.5 mm × 244 mm) of a commercially available laptop (Surface Laptop 3, Microsoft, Redmond, WA). The area of eye capture was 35 cm × 30 cm at 65 cm distance. Eye movement analyses were conducted automatically by the eye tracker based on the combined assessment of corneal reflection and pupillary contrast to the white sclera. The movement pattern is recorded as x and y values over time.

To ensure a standardized study environment, all volunteers were exposed to the same set of images in the same room, under identical light and seating conditions. Volunteers were asked to sit upright on a chair with a fixed backrest, at a distance of 45 cm to the screen. Before visual stimulus exposure, a nine-point calibration was conducted to ensure consistency throughout the eye movement analyses.

Visual Stimulus Presented

A total of 10 facial images were presented to the 58 study volunteers for the duration of 6 seconds each (= image exposure interval). Between images, participants were presented with a white screen for 2 seconds, to allow for gaze relaxation. Of the 10 displayed images, five images showed patients before lower eyelid blepharoplasty (**Fig. 1**) and the other five images showed the same set of patients 1 year after their surgical intervention (**Fig. 2**; **Figs. 3** and **4**). The presented preoperative and postoperative images were displayed in a randomized sequence to accommodate for learners' bias. A stable eye fixation was defined as a constant eye fixation for the duration of at least 0.08 seconds.

All performed surgical procedures followed standard lower eyelid blepharoplasty guidelines without specific modifications. Images were transferred for the purposes of this study to a research center following patient informed consent.

Data Analysis

Eye movement pattern analysis
Data were analyzed according to a previously published protocol.[13] In brief, the following variables were captured:

- Time until first fixation (interval between initial display of the image and the first stable eye fixation)
- Time of fixation (duration of a stable eye fixation within the time of visual stimulus exposure = 6 seconds)

All parameters captured were stratified by areas of visual interest: periorbital, nose, perioral.

Statistical analysis
The data were normally distributed, as assessed by Shapiro-Wilk test ($P > .05$). Differences of the total time of fixation and time until first fixation between volunteers with and without plastic surgical background were calculated using Student t test. Differences between facial region were calculated by analysis of variance with post hoc Tukey testing. All calculations were performed using SPSS Statistics version 26 (IBM, Armonk, NY) and results were considered statistically significant at a probability level of less than or equal to 0.05 to guide conclusions.

RESULTS
General Findings

Overall, there was a statistically significant difference in the eye movement pattern between volunteers with and without plastic surgery background ($P < .004$).

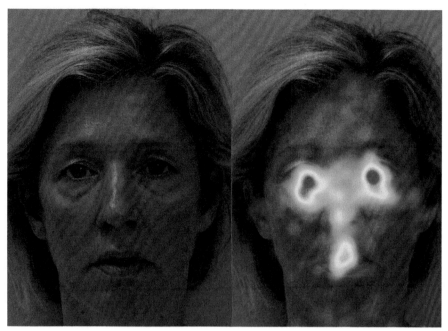

Fig. 1. Frontal view showing the preoperative image on the left and the superimposed average gaze pattern of the observers on the right.

Sequence of Fixation

Randomized visual stimulus exposure revealed that in the preoperative images volunteers first focused on the periorbital region with 0.81 (0.9) seconds, followed by the nose with 1.03 (1.4) seconds and by the perioral region with 2.17 (1.4) seconds ($P < .001$). In the postoperative images, the sequence of fixation was first the nose with 0.96 (1.3) seconds followed by the periorbital regions with 1.84 (0.99) seconds and by the perioral region with 2.18 (1.4) seconds ($P < .001$).

Comparing the time to first fixation between the preoperative and postoperative images showed that the time for the perioral region ($P = .941$) and the time for the nose ($P = .516$) did not change

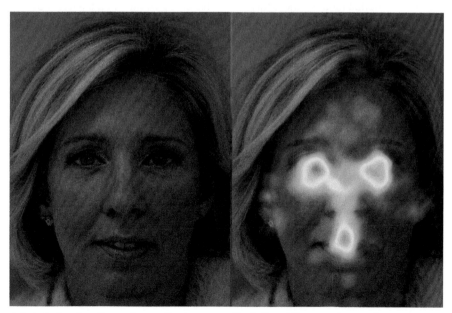

Fig. 2. Frontal view showing the postoperative image on the left and the superimposed average gaze pattern of the observers on the right. Note the decrease of intensity in the periorbital region.

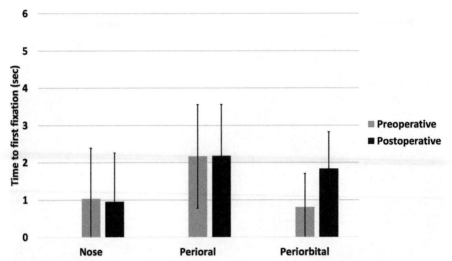

Fig. 3. Bar graph showing the mean time to fixation for the respective facial regions (periorbital, perioral, and nose) when looking at the preoperative and the postoperative images.

on a statistically significant level. However, the time to first fixation statistically significantly increased from preoperative to postoperative for the periorbital region (P < .001 from 0.81 seconds to 1.84 seconds).

Total Duration of Fixation

The total time volunteers spent on inspecting each of the three facial regions of interest during the 6-second image exposure interval was for images showing preoperative faces 0.72 (0.5) seconds for the perioral region, 0.75 (0.6) seconds for the nose, and 2.22 (0.7) seconds for the periorbital region (P < .001). The duration of stable eye fixation

was for images showing postoperative facial images 0.74 (0.5) seconds for the perioral region, 0.85 (0.7) seconds for the nose, and 1.26 (0.6) seconds for the periorbital region (P < .001).

These durations indicate that there was no statistically significant change following surgery for the perioral region (P = .689) and for the nose (P = .090). However, the periorbital region duration statistically significantly reduced from 2.22 seconds to 1.26 seconds (P < .001).

DISCUSSION

This study investigated the eye movement pattern of 58 volunteers when looking at randomized

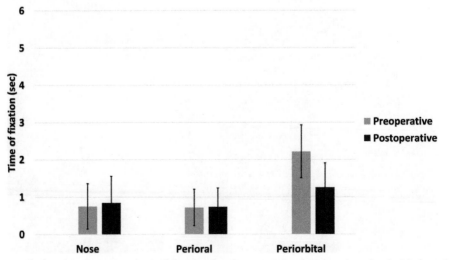

Fig. 4. Bar graph showing the mean time of fixation for the respective facial regions (periorbital, perioral, and nose) when looking at the preoperative and the postoperative images.

preoperative and postoperative images of a total of five patients following lower eyelid blepharoplasty. The results revealed that the sequence of facial recognition before surgery was periorbital-nose-perioral, whereas following surgery the sequence was nose-periorbital-perioral. The time until the first stable eye fixation was detected by the eye tracking device did, however, not defer between the nose (pre vs post: 1.03 vs 0.96 seconds) and the perioral region (2.17 vs 2.18 seconds) on a statistically significant level ($P = .516$ for nose and $P = .941$ for perioral). This is in line with the setup of the study because no other facial intervention was performed on the patients except lower eyelid blepharoplasty and that influenced the appearance of the periorbital region only. The time until first fixation changed on a statistically significant level with 0.81 versus 1.84 seconds from the presurgical to the postsurgical facial image for the periorbital region, indicating an increase in the interval between initial image display and stable eye fixation. The increase in time most likely indicates a decrease in attraction toward an area that was perceived by the inspecting volunteers as less pleasing. Because it might seem counterintuitive to be less attracted to an area that underwent surgical attention (and has improved following the procedure), the results seem plausible when incorporating the concept of "internal representation of beauty." This concept is based on the assumption that beauty is a predefined internal status that the individual tries to find in objects or facial features inspected. Because this status is conditioned by the socioethnocultural development of the individual it is understandable that beauty varies among cultures and individuals and can change throughout professional or cultural development. Objects or facial features that match into that predefined concept of beauty require less attention by the individual to be perceived or processed because the visual stimulus fits into the preconditioned internal image of beauty. On the contrary, objects that do not match into that predefined concept of beauty do require more attention and effort to be perceived and understood because of the mismatch between the internal status of beauty and external visual stimulus; this might be perceived by the individual as less beautiful.[10,11]

Translating this concept of internal representation of beauty into the data of this study, it is confirmed that the preoperative image showing the periorbital region was inspected statistically significantly faster than the postoperative image; this is in line with the concept presented. Because the other facial regions did not change from the preintervention to the postintervention image there was no statistically relevant change in the time of first fixation.

Investigating the duration of stable eye fixations (longer than 0.08 seconds) during the 6-second image exposure interval revealed that there was no statistically relevant change in the duration for viewing the nose or the perioral region. However, the duration for viewing the periorbital region statistically significantly reduced from 2.22 seconds to 1.26 seconds ($P < .001$). This is understood as the need for less internal processing of viewing a beautiful facial feature because it matches more the internal standard of beauty. The other facial regions did not require the volunteers to alter their eye movement pattern because no change occurred between the preinterventional and the postinterventional image.

When analyzing the difference between surgical experience of the volunteers (n = 12 [20.7%] were plastic surgeons and n = 46 [79.3%] were without medical background) the concept of the internal standard of beauty was repeatedly supported: volunteers with plastic surgery background had a shorter time to first fixation and a longer duration of visual stimulus inspection; this was similar in trend for the preoperative and the postoperative images. This is interpreted as the increased attention of the experienced observer toward an aesthetically less pleasing facial feature compared with the nonexperienced observer. Volunteers with plastic surgical background perceived those areas as potentially less beautiful because of their altered internal representation of beauty and facial features caught quicker their attention and they needed longer time to process the image presented.[10]

This study is not free of limitations. The 58 volunteers were altogether of White ethnicity as were the preoperative and postoperative images of the patients used as visual stimulus. It could be speculated that the aesthetic perception would be different if the patients and/or the volunteers would be of African-American or Asian ethnicity. Future studies need investigate ethnic influences on eye movement pattern.

Focusing on the sequence of facial recognition during image exposure it can be stated that based on the results presented herein a modular facial inspection approach is conducted by the volunteers included in this investigation. Certain facial features were viewed, such as the nose, mouth, and eyes, but the sequence altered depending on the aesthetic liking of the observer. The eyes or the periorbital region were not inspected first; the time until eye movements had a stable eye fixation varied based on the surgical status of the patient displayed. A less aesthetically pleasing facial feature was inspected first (periorbital preoperative image) but once this mismatch was improved (in the present study because of surgery) the periorbital region was not inspected first anymore. It is hypothesized that there might be a natural sequence of facial feature recognition, but this sequence might be influenced by the internal representation of beauty of the observer. A less aesthetically pleasing facial feature might "disrupt" the natural sequence of facial feature recognition and could influence therefore the direction of attention during facial inspection. However, the conducted study is limited in its power to conclusively support the assumptions made and future studies need to elaborate on the findings presented herein.

SUMMARY

This eye tracking analysis–based study revealed that the sequence of facial feature recognition is influenced by the aesthetic liking of the observer and that alteration to facial features influences the sequence of facial feature recognition. The eye movement pattern, however, seems to follow the internal representation of beauty where aesthetically pleasing facial features are observed later during first image exposure and are viewed shorter during a visual stimulus exposure interval.

CLINICS CARE POINTS

The sequence of facial feature recognition is influenced by the aesthetic liking of the observerIteration to facial features influences the sequence of facial feature recognition aesthetically pleasing facial features are observed later during first image exposure and are viewed shorter during a visual stimulus exposure interval.

REFERENCES

1. International Society of Aesthetic Plastic Surgeons. ISAPS international survey on aesthetic/cosmetic procedures performed in 2017 2019. Available at. https://www.isaps.org/wp-content/uploads/2019/03/ ISAPS_2017_International_Study_Cosmetic_Procedures_ NEW.pdf. Accessed date May 6, 2019.
2. Kruglikov I, Trujillo O, Kristen Q, et al. The facial adipose tissue: a revision. Facial Plast Surg 2016; 32(06):671–82.
3. Cotofana S, Schenck TL, Trevidic P, et al. Midface: clinical anatomy and regional approaches with injectable fillers. Plast Reconstr Surg 2015;136: 219S–34S.
4. Cotofana S, Gotkin RH, Frank K, et al. The functional anatomy of the deep facial fat compartments: a detailed imaging-based investigation. Plast Reconstr Surg 2019;143(1):53–63.
5. Cotofana S, Gotkin RH, Ascher B, et al. Calvarial volume loss and facial aging: a computed tomographic (CT)-based study. Aesthet Surg J 2018;38(10): 1043–51.
6. Frank K, Gotkin RH, Pavicic T, et al. Age and gender differences of the frontal bone: a computed tomographic (CT)-based study. Aesthet Surg J 2018; 39(7):699–710.
7. Cotofana S, Gotkin RH, Morozov SP, et al. The relationship between bone remodeling and the clockwise rotation of the facial skeleton: a computed tomography imaging based evaluation. Plast Reconstr Surg 2018;142(6):1447–54.
8. Schenck TL, Koban KC, Schlattau A, et al. The functional anatomy of the superficial fat compartments of the face: a detailed imaging study. Plast Reconstr Surg 2018;141(6):1351–9.
9. Mojallal A, Cotofana S. Anatomy of lower eyelid and eyelid–cheek junction. Ann Chir Plast Esthétique 2017;62(5):365–74.
10. Cai LZ, Paro JAM, Lee GK, et al. Where do we look? Assessing gaze patterns in breast reconstructive surgery with eye-tracking technology. Plast Reconstr Surg 2018;141(3):331E–40E.
11. Jansen A, Nederkoorn C, Mulkens S. Selective visual attention for ugly and beautiful body parts in eating disorders. Behav Res Ther 2005;43(2): 183–96.
12. WMA Declaration of Helsinki – ethical principles for medical research involving human subjects – WMA – the World Medical Association. Available at. https://www.wma.net/policies-post/wma-declaration-of-helsinki-ethical-principles-for-medical-research-involving-human-subjects/. Accessed August 5, 2018.
13. Frank K, Moellhoff N, Swift A, et al. In search of the most attractive lip-proportions and lip-volume: an eye tracking- and survey-based investigation. Plast Reconstr Surg.; In Print.

Printed and bound by CPI Group (UK) Ltd, Croydon, CR0 4YY

08/05/2025

01864704-0017